MY STORY

my story

A PHOTOGRAPHIC ESSAY ON LIFE WITH MULTIPLE SCLEROSIS

Amelia Davis

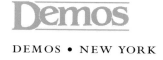

DEMOS • NEW YORK

Demos Medical Publishing, Inc. 386 Park Avenue South,
New York, NY 10016, USA

Library of Congress Cataloging-in-Publication Data
Davis, Amelia, 1968–
  My story : a photographic essay of life with multiple sclerosis
/ Amelia Davis.
      p. cm.
  ISBN 1-932603-01-8 (pbk.)
  1. Multiple sclerosis—Patients—Biography. 2. Multiple
sclerosis—Patients—Biography—Pictorial works. I. Title.
  RC377.D377 2004
  362.196'834'0092—dc22
                              2003017020

Designed and typeset by Gopa & Ted2, Inc.

Made in the United States of America

For Bonita

My caregiver, My strength. Thank you.

Contents

Foreword

PEOPLE OFTEN THINK that a diagnosis of multiple sclerosis is the end of their ability to live a normal life. By watching my husband Richard, I know this isn't true. MS is simply the next chapter. Together we have found there is always something new to discover, even if it's just the dawn of a new day.

In a society where the disabled are often forgotten and left behind, it is important to remember that physical disability is just that—a physical condition. Beyond the body, there is the mind, hungry for knowledge and wisdom. And beyond the mind there is the need for love.

Richard has shown me that the obstacles of physical limitation are challenges that we must circumvent and not surrender to. Despite it all, we continue to build our lives and have learned that joy lies in the simple things.

Because MS dances on different stages, it is often difficult to address. While one person struggles with fatigue, another battles cognitive problems. It is not in the differences that those with MS find common ground; it's in the certainty that the emotional battles can be fought and won with courage and commitment. It takes a dedication to one's own growth and the certainty that life can be lived with grace, humor, substance and fortitude no matter what the adversity we face as human beings.

People often ask how Richard is doing. Like anyone who lives with MS, there are good days and bad days. But I have found that even the bad days are a blessing. There is always something to appreciate when you open your eyes and look around you.

Richard and I are proud to be a part of this book. These are the smiles, the statures and the eyes of MS. They look out from the page to remind you that no matter the face that MS wears, behind the glance there is a whole person looking back at you.

Jennifer Lee Pryor

Preface

FIVE YEARS AGO, just two months before my thirtieth birthday I was diagnosed with multiple sclerosis (MS). I had no idea what it was. I thought I was too young to be diagnosed with a chronic illness. How could this be?

It wasn't until I did my own research that I found out that all of my preconceived ideas about what MS was and looked like were wrong. At that point, I realized there was a real need for a photographic book about people living with this disorder. The first year I was diagnosed with MS I was so sick that I rarely left my bed. I began to rely on the emotional and financial support of my partner and caregiver. As a result of this experience, my desire was to not only show the public what people living with MS looked and felt like, but also to portray the important role that caregivers and family members play in the life of a person living with this disease.

When a disease is represented to the public, its many different faces are often left out. MS does not discriminate. It affects people of all ages, races and backgrounds. Some people such as myself require no aid at all; some use canes, some use motorized scooters, while others use wheelchairs. On the outside, many people with MS—including myself—look perfectly healthy. No one would ever know that we are fighting an inward battle with our own bodies. This is the reality of MS. MS does not always have the same outcome for everyone and sometimes it is a difficult fate to accept. But, by confronting reality and looking at it straight on, we who live with MS can come together and recognize each other's challenges and help push away the stereotypes society has about this disease.

One of the most important messages conveyed through this book is to take control of MS before it controls you. There are drugs and other therapies that can make a difference. No specific therapy is right for everyone. So choose one that works best for you and your lifestyle. Through a wide variety of innovative and often inspirational techniques, everyone in this book has taken control of his or her life in some way.

Many major drug companies have come together to show their support for this book, and to help educate the public, as well as people living with MS. What an amazing commitment!

Through my journey I have met some truly exceptional human beings. They have both inspired and humbled me. They have taught me to celebrate life no matter what it may deal you. I hope we can all learn from them.

Acknowledgments

First, I would like to thank all the people featured in this book who welcomed me into their lives and have become my friends. You all are extraordinary human beings.

Dave Hultman played an instrumental role in getting funding for this book and making it a reality.

The Northern California Chapter of the National Multiple Sclerosis Society provided help in bringing this book to completion. Special thanks go to Terence Keane and Mary Lou Torre.

Special thanks go to the following people from the different drug companies who rallied for this book and me: Cindy North and Jeanine O' Kane from Berlex, Jennifer Westphal from Fleishman-Hillard Inc./ Teva, Jeff McLaughlin from Spectrum Science / Biogen, and Lyndi Hersch from Serono. Thanks as well to Liz Pendergast and the Champions of Courage.

Printing of this book was undertaken, in part, with a grant from Berlex.

Andrew Blauner, my agent, once again understood the importance and need for this book. Thank you for believing in my work. Dr. Diana M. Schneider, Publisher of Demos, knew how much this book was needed. She welcomed it and never looked back.

When I was trying to find a publisher, Margot Russell jumped in and found Demos. Kathleen Wilson provided endless help and friendship. Thank you for convincing funders that this book is a worthwhile and invaluable tool. Special thanks go to MSWorld for its support.

I am grateful to Elizabeth Davis, my sister, for her constant support and to my niece, Madeleine Isabelle, for adding a ray of light into my life.

Jim Marshall offered unquestioning help and support. I am grateful for his friendship.

Kirk Anspach not only did all the printing of my photographs, but also supplied encouragement and support of my work.

And finally, Bonita—caregiver, friend, guide, assistant/editor, partner in life, and without a doubt the most caring and talented person I have ever known. Thank you for showing me that tomorrow is always a new day.

This book could not have been completed without the generous financial contributions of the following organizations and individuals

CORPORATE AND FOUNDATION CONTRIBUTORS

Champions of Courage, an independant organization sponsored by Berlex

Biogen

Teva Neuroscience

Serono

www.msworld.org

INDIVIDUAL CONTRIBUTORS

Paul Alotta

Erika and Arthur Andreas

Dr. Jay Azling

Greg Block

Cynthia Brattesani, DDS

Janice Brouhard

Robert L. Brown
and Kirstin Hoefer

Dr. and Mrs. Gavin Carr

Patrick Convey
and Edward Barlow

Marianne Clark

Mr. and Mrs. Ian Davidson

Anne (Treglia)
and Gus Emmick, MD

Michal and Richard Feder

Helen Greenwood

Dr. William Hawthorne
and Edwin M. Hacker

Florence and Jim Hitchcock

Jeff Hultman

Antoine and Tracy Kemper

Phoebe Liebig

Kenneth Leibler,
Boston Stock Exchange

Viola Lucero

Richard Lynch

William and Emily Moran

Elizabeth Moreton

J. William Morris III

Bill and Nancy Newmeyer

Doug and Paige Nicholson

Anne Overton

Julie Overton

Corinne and Robert Powers

Charles Richards

Nancy and R. C. Ribak

David Evans Rosedahl

Bill Ryan

ABN AMRO Sage

Harriet Schley

Betty Cobey Senescu

Ken and Linda Slavin

Morris S. Smith Foundation

Richard and Lucille Treglia

Thomas and Delinda Trowbridge

Mr. and Mrs. Don Whitaker

Sarah and Mark Williamson

Robert Yahng

The Stories

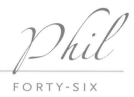

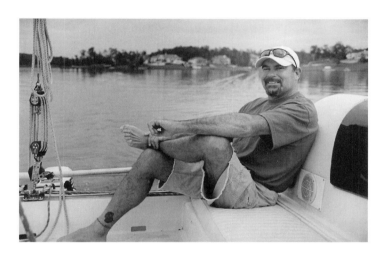

I HAD JUST RETURNED to the dock on a beautiful June afternoon in 1994 after a physically demanding set of water ski jumps. On one jump I fell pretty hard but finished the set and called it a day. Later that week I noticed a slight numbness or tingling sensation in my left leg. I attributed it to the fall and thought I had better take it easy for awhile. However, the feeling did not go away and in fact got worse. That's when I knew something wasn't right.

I've always been a water sports lover. The year before I was diagnosed with MS I had coached the United States Disabled Water Ski Team to the country's first overall gold medal. I have devoted my career to work in therapeutic recreation and can remember as far back as elementary school that this was the direction I wanted my life to take. It was this calling that propelled me to begin a program called Adaptive Aquatics, one of the first nonprofit water skiing programs for people with disabilities. The program, begun in 1980, was staffed entirely by volunteers, and consisted of weekend clinics in the South where those with physical and mental disabilities would be provided with the opportunity to experience adaptive water skiing. My work with disabled individ-

3

uals has allowed me to become associated with some of the most incredible and inspirational people one could ever hope to meet.

I view my diagnosis more as irony than anything else. After fifteen years of working in the field of therapeutic recreation, I was told I had a debilitating disease myself. I worried that my love for water sports, particularly water skiing, might be in jeopardy due to the fatigue and the heat related problems associated with MS. But life is all about changes (especially for those with MS), so I shifted my focus from the very physical sport of water skiing to the less demanding (at least on the legs) sport of sailing. This change put an end to the fast-paced 10-12 hour days of instructing ski clinics to the more leisurely paced sport of sailing.

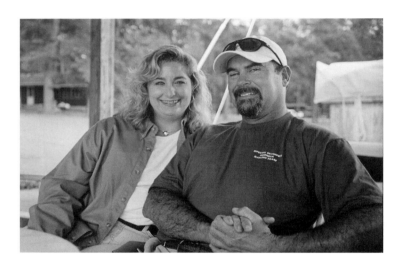

So how do I feel now after having MS for eight years? I feel very fortunate to have a wonderful neurologist to help guide me; thankful for the new medications to control the disease and its symptoms, and blessed to be surrounded by positive friends and family. My sixteen-year-old son, Drew, who survived childhood cancer, has been a constant inspiration. And since this book is dedicated to those with MS and their care providers, I must make special mention of Kristin: my girlfriend, care provider, and cheerleader. She has been with me through the ups and downs of the past seven years. It would be difficult without her.

I don't have time to be down. I am always having too much fun. Life is great and I am not going to let MS get in the way of living mine to the fullest.

KRISTIN

A small, framed print of a sailboat hangs on the bathroom wall and reads:
"We can not direct the wind, but we can adjust our sails." It is this simple, yet powerful phrase which guides our life everyday.

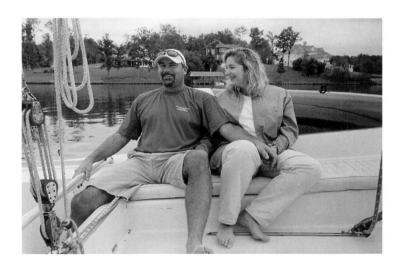

Phil had already been diagnosed with MS when I met him in 1995. I was working for a YWCA at the time and he would bring a group of Special Olympic athletes in to train on a regular basis as part of his job as Adaptive Program Coordinator for our local parks and recreation department. Besides his broad grin and sparkling eyes, it was his optimistic view of life which immediately attracted me to him.

I joined Phil as a volunteer for his adaptive water skiing program that year. We traveled around the South most weekends for several summers thereafter providing those incredibly inspirational water skiing clinics. The smile on the faces of the participants after each triumphant ski run was indescribable. Phil loved doing the clinics, but it began to take longer and longer for him to overcome the physical exhaustion afterwards. Ten and twelve hour days in the sun were just too much. In 1999, it was time to adjust his sails. Many in Phil's position might have viewed this as a great loss, something that MS took away. But he saw it as an opportunity to begin something else new and just as rewarding. While bittersweet, it was with great pride that he turned his work over to a dear friend and early participant of the program. Today, the organization is flourishing and Phil still stays involved as a consultant.

Some may be hesitant to enter into a relationship with a person who has a debilitating disease like MS. There is no doubt that it can be difficult. It adds another layer of complexity to issues that need to be communicated and understood. But by and far the most important element in our relationship is the power of the positive. The glass is never half-empty; it's always half full. In life as in sailing, every day is a just a matter of determining which way the wind is blowing and we trim our sails accordingly.

Since 1999, Phil's attention has been devoted to building a sailing program for people with disabilities. This year's adventures will take him to Ireland for the sailing portion of the Special Olympic World Games. I am currently learning to sail under his direction as well, but perhaps he has already taught me the most important lesson of all; you cannot direct the wind but you *can* adjust your sails.

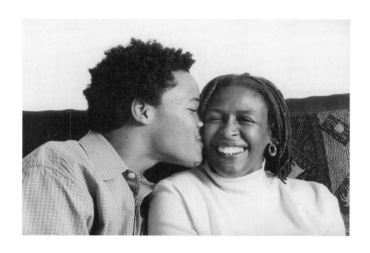

IN 1993 I HAD ARTHROSCOPIC SUR-GERY on my knee for what at the time was joint discomfort. When the healing process took longer than expected a relative suggested I get another opinion. Because she was a nurse I took her along as we visited an orthopedic specialist at her place of employment. Upon examination the doctor stated that the problem wasn't my knee but rather something neurologic; he then recommended I undergo further tests, as the diagnosis could be a brain tumor or MS.

Because I worked at Oregon Health Sciences University I was able to get in immediately for further tests and at the end of two weeks I received the answer—multiple sclerosis. Having not known anyone with this disease, nor being in any way familiar with its ramifications, I plunged myself into study of how it would impact my future.

Being a divorced parent of a then eight-year-old child, I worried how this diagnosis would impact our lives and most importantly our future. It's been ten years now and that eight-year-old is now about to graduate from high school. I've since retired from my job and many other milestones have occurred in between.

7

I can say that as we've embraced MS and not let it "have us" our life has been the better for it. I went from walking with a gait, to using a cane, from the cane to a walker, and most recently received a motorized scooter for better mobility. Each phase has brought with it a sense of loss but we've made the adjustments and continued to be participants in life.

I had wondered what I would do with myself after retiring at such a young age. While I was thankful for my twenty years of employment at the University and the retirement benefit that accompanied my leaving, I was uncertain about my next step and where I would find value. I'm

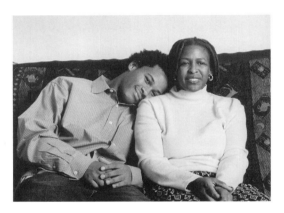 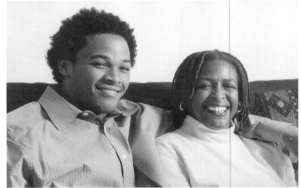

happy to say that I lead a full life and depending on the day am involved in activities such as water exercise at the local pool, leading a women's bible group at my church, participating in a writing workshop with other members of the MS community, or a myriad of other activities that bring me joy and strength.

I've learned that while life indeed can throw us curves, it's our reaction to those curves that define who we are and help us build character. Of my accomplishments I'm most proud of my son, Bobby, a young man whose life was forever changed by the two letters MS. He has grown into a caring, compassionate person and largely because of the uncertainty this disease has brought into his life, has gained the capacity to adapt and take life by the horns.

As I've observed him assisting others who are similarly disabled or taking that extra time with children to listen to and attend to their needs, I say, "thank you, MS, you've made us both better people and helped us to see the important things in life."

Bobby

I was eight years old when my mom was diagnosed with MS. This diagnosis was the beginning of many changes in my life, some big and some small. The big changes included becoming more responsible at a younger age and having to look out for something greater than myself. My to-do list became bigger, too, as my mom became increasingly incapable of doing things. Mowing the lawn and taking out the garbage became my job. Because my mom and my dad had divorced three years earlier, it was just she and I; add to that this disease and both our worlds changed dramatically.

In many ways I feel somewhat cheated, as because of my mom's MS I had to act "grown up" at such a young age and forgo the carefree years of just being a young boy. The resentment I have felt from this has sometimes inappropriately been directed at my mom. I've since realized it's not her, rather the disease that robbed us both and caused me anxiety.

I have learned a lot of things in these ten years of living with this disease. One of the main lessons is that no matter how bad life seems there is always someone worse off than you. If they can get up and stay in the game of life, then those of us who are "healthy" have little excuse. For that type of inspiration I thank MS and my mom.

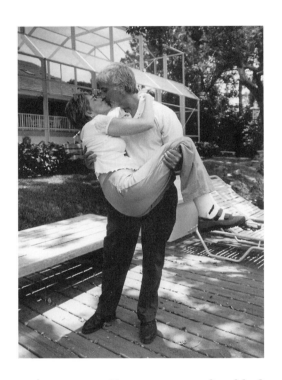

FIFTEEN YEARS AGO, while at a monthly appointment with my neurologist, he commented that I was a lucky girl. Given that I had hobbled into his office on a cane while other patients waited in wheelchairs, I assumed he was referring to my physical well-being. After graduating to a wheelchair many years later, I understand that he was referring to my husband, Ken—who is my caregiver, and to the quality of our marital relationship. Twenty-three years of marriage speaks for itself; I am indeed a lucky girl.

Multiple sclerosis is an exceptionally selfish disease. It has challenged my courage, my confidence and my career. Facing an unpredictable future is much like making a wish and flipping over an eight ball! Being a psychotherapist by trade, I know how to advise and respond to others, but early on, anger, denial and diversion served me well. For many years, most people did not know I had MS, and those that knew me would always say, "you look really good." Little did they know I was hiding numbness, spasticity, and personal anguish.

In 1989, I developed a private practice of my own, counseling Adult Children of Alcoholics. I had earned a master's degree in Rehabilitation Counseling and for several years, I had my "fifteen minutes of fame." However, the fatigue from my progressing multiple sclerosis made even part-time work difficult.

In 1998, my husband and I moved to Florida, where I presently reside. My worst nightmare played out right before my eyes when I progressed from using a cane, to a walker, and finally to a wheelchair. I've always been a strong-willed fighter so, feeling that I had nothing to lose and everything to gain, I began a customized exercise program. My personal trainer devised a comprehensive workout program consisting of strength training, punch-boxing, swimming and stretching. This has significantly increased my ability to function independently with the laborious tasks of personal care and day-to-day activities. I have supplemented these activities with new medications, which have been highly effective in slowing the progress of my MS.

After our relocation, a key goal was to keep my condition from worsening. However, the piece of the puzzle still not in place for me has been resuming the passion I once had for helping others to help themselves. I hope to work online with clients in a "Dear Abby" fashion where concerns and questions are discussed via e-mail.

Although I need to use a wheelchair, I am stronger both in body and mind. In addition, I receive a weekly massage. Exercise paired with massage is the secret ingredient to my success. They have improved my circulation, developed tone and body definition, and made the transfer of my own body weight no longer a struggle. If attitude is everything, my mission is to be fit and first in line when a cure rolls around.

I have always been a firm believer that everything in life happens for a reason. I am forever changed because of MS and truthfully, I like the new me. While multiple sclerosis limits my mobility, it has offered me the unique opportunity to work with all my caregivers. Their expertise, encouragement, friendship and love have restored what MS has taken away. I am honored to call these skilled, sincere, supportive and caring individuals my family.

Kenny, my husband, daily caregiver, and best friend, has always focused his life around me. Thank you for your endless patience, love, dedication and for choosing to stay. You are the reason I am here. I am loved and very lucky! On good days, I hope you feel the same.

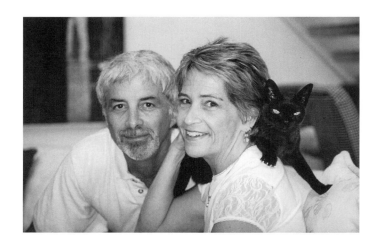

KENNY

I first heard the words "multiple sclerosis" during a doctor's appointment for my wife, Linda. She had been experiencing numbness in her extremities, much like symptoms she had experienced three years before. Linda called to schedule an appointment with her neurologist, but since he was away, his associate conducted the examination. Unaware that the diagnosis of multiple sclerosis had not been mentioned to us, the doctor casually began discussing Linda's condition in reference to the disease. We sat there for a few minutes in a daze. I remember leaving the examination room and having to lean against the corridor wall to keep my legs from collapsing underneath me.

During the proceeding months, we tried to learn as much as we could about multiple sclerosis. Linda's symptoms up to that point were mild and the doctor suggested that was a positive sign. Perhaps the course of the disease would be mild as well. For both of us, the uncertainty of the future was the hardest thing to cope with.

Over time, Linda's symptoms worsened and it became apparent that our original marital roles must change. Chronic fatigue and weakness left Linda with diminished ability to complete the daily routine she had always taken for granted. I found myself having to assume some of her responsibilities as well as my own. Frequent doctor visits, weekly prescription runs, and trying to sched-ule my work around illness-related problems became routine. Preparing meals and cleaning up, something we had always shared, now became my sole responsibility. Without the help of family members, caring for Linda and trying to buoy her spirits was to be my job alone.

From time to time, caring for Linda seemed overwhelming. I found it necessary to take time out for myself and to delegate responsibility to outside professionals. To make life easier, we relo-cated to a warmer climate. Having to leave good friends behind and start a new life was difficult.

It has been fifteen years since Linda's diagnosis. We've overcome many obstacles but with the help and support of doctors, friends and professionals, we've made a life. Life with MS is tough at best; but with the conviction to make it work, together we've achieved our goal. It's a good life after all!

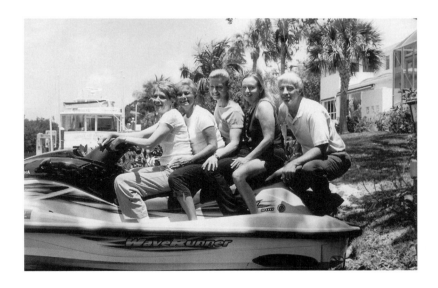

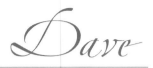

Dave

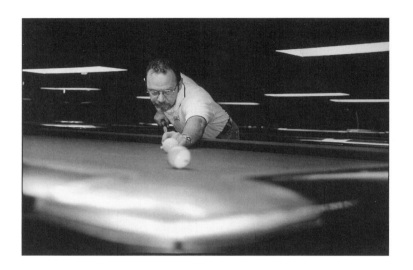

FORTY-NINE

I HAD BEEN A HORSESHOER by trade for more then ten years (and loving it), when it started getting progressively more difficult to perform my job due to fatigue and muscle spasms. I had always been in good shape and really identified myself with my work. After struggling for a few years I retired from my trade with secret guilty feelings. I seemed to have become burned out and lazy. Somehow I was no longer the hard-working person I had envisioned myself to be. It would be several years before a diagnosis of multiple sclerosis would put a rest to this nagging self-doubt.

It took quite a while but I have learned many things about life and about myself since my diagnosis. I am the same person whether I can still shoe horses or not—if I can't do that, I can still do something else. Finding something you can do that you love helps you feel better physically, mentally, and emotionally. Be flexible, have goals, and remember that certain forces are beyond everyone's control. We need to fight back to find out what we can do and can't do. If there is something we can't do we must adjust and readjust if necessary. One of the reasons I consider myself lucky is because I believe in myself and have not quit trying to make things happen. This is the only life I have. My real job is to continue to grow personally and spiritually, to love more and to enjoy myself along the way. No disease can take my real job away. Everyone has limitations, and we can choose to focus either on what we can do or on what we can't do. One helps us in our real job and one does not, but it's our choice.

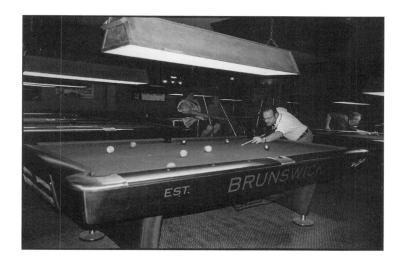

Fighting back for me has meant a lot of things. Redoubling my efforts at my childhood love for competitive pool has been key as well as taking advantage of the medical interventions available. It has also been important to accept help from others when necessary and to come to terms with the reality that I have limitations, just like everyone else. Teaching others—I'm the House Pro at two pool halls—is also a way in which I fight back. It takes me away from worrying about my own problems, which can cause a self-centered spiraling into depression. Competing against "healthy" individuals on an even par has also been helpful even when I lose a match. After all, I have still won a small battle against MS! Worrying is a waste of energy. What's really lacking right now, at this very instant?

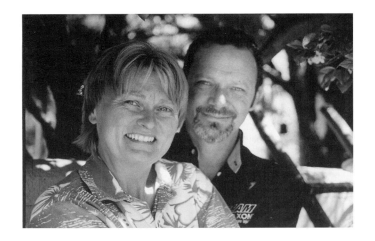

I don't want to sound like I have everything figured out. I have my share of bad days. My wife Geni will attest to that. But I'm working on it. When I first went to the doctor I was told that I either had MS or an inoperable tumor in my spine. I was crushed and couldn't decide which to hope for. The truth is I was leaning toward the tumor. Both possibilities appeared to be death sentences—one relatively short and one long and drawn out. Yet the first impressions we have about some things can be misleading.

I guess the main lesson I have learned from this is that we should never stop trying to make the most of our life. Here I am three years later living out a childhood dream of being a touring pool player. How cool is that?

Geni

Multiple sclerosis. Every so often it has this way of reminding you. Sometimes just little reminders like numbness, itching, blurry vision and fatigue. Other times big stuff like anger and depression. Multiple sclerosis has lots of tricks.

For me the very hardest part is the fear. That constant little nag in my stomach. At first I passed it off on world events, then stress at work and lots of other guesses. Finally, I figured it out. I'm scared of MS all the time. I'm scared for me, I'm scared for David and I'm scared for us. It never goes away.

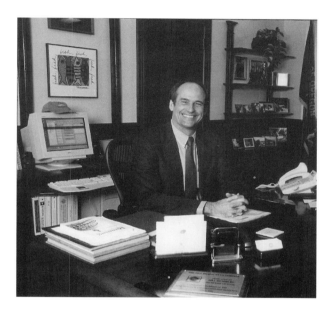

A LITTLE OVER TWENTY YEARS AGO, I was diagnosed with multiple sclerosis. It was 1980 and I was running in my very first political campaign for the Oregon House of Representatives.

During the campaign, I started noticing that my eyes were crossing. I went to an optometrist, who told me, "You've either got a brain tumor or multiple sclerosis." He referred me to a neurologist—and I never thought I'd say this, but I was pretty thrilled when he told me a few months later that I had MS, and not a brain tumor!

I was only a few months into my very first session in the Oregon Legislature. I remember wondering what the diagnosis meant for my future. Could I have MS and be a successful elected official?

I knew that I had the drive and the dreams to get me there—I never questioned that—but I worried that people's perception of the disease might stand in my way. I worried that voters would be distracted by the slight limp and not notice that I was a dedicated, passionate and energetic leader.

17

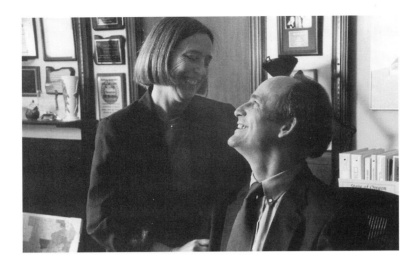

Fortunately, that hasn't been the case. After serving as a state representative, I went on to serve the people of Oregon as a state senator, senate president and now secretary of state.

When I was running my campaign for election, someone asked me if I thought having MS would keep me from winning. I told them that thankfully, this was a political race, not a foot race. I wasn't too sure I'd win a foot race, but I felt pretty good about the political one.

There are lots of ways to do a job. And just as each of us has our own challenges, so too do each of us have our own strengths. I face having multiple sclerosis. When people think of leaders, they don't usually think of people with MS—but that doesn't mean that I can't be a leader and also have MS. It just means I have to make a few accommodations.

When voters look at me, yes, they probably notice that I walk a little funny. They probably see that I have to lean on the railing when I walk upstairs and that I sit down during long speeches—but they also see that I am energized by hard work, that serving the people of Oregon is what keeps me happy, motivated and healthy.

In fact, after I finished serving a lengthy and contentious term as senate president, my doctor said he had never seen me looking and feeling so good.

My ability to walk up and down stairs has nothing to do with my ability to serve as a leader—and the simple reality is that having MS doesn't keep me from doing the job that Oregon's voters elected me to do with energy and commitment.

I think it's good for Oregon to have leaders that reflect the communities they serve—and those communities include people of different races, genders, orientations and abilities. Hiding my disease from my supporters or feeling ashamed of my disability just doesn't work for me. What does work is being up front with folks, facing the disease head-on, and tackling each new day with energy, hope and humor—and you know what? I think that philosophy has kept me healthier than any treatment alone ever could.

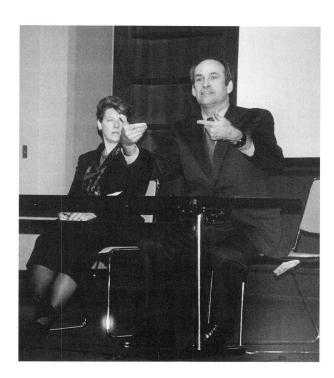

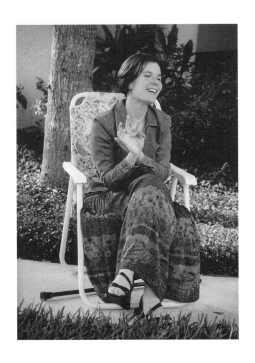

I WAS DIAGNOSED with multiple sclerosis one month after my twenty-fourth birthday. At the time I was actually relieved just to know what was happening to me.

A few months earlier, my new husband and I had to return a week early from "the trip of a lifetime" to Australia and New Zealand. While on this vacation, I had my first exacerbation—a bad one. It got to the point where I couldn't feel my body from the chest down, and at the time, even the doctors didn't have a clue as to what was going on. They suggested that I might have a rapidly-growing tumor or blood clot on my spinal cord—both of which would immediately need to be ruled out with an MRI before I could even safely leave the country. After finding out there was no tumor or clot, and given the green light to return home, we left Australia, having never set foot in New Zealand.

My husband Jonathan and I had planned to try to start a family after our trip. Obviously, we had no idea that we would be returning home under these circumstances! We decided to postpone our plans until we could find out what was going on. It was a difficult time, as we desperately wanted to proceed with our lives.

After we returned to the States, and following a course of IV-steroid treatment, I was actually much better—but we still didn't know what was the matter. I was devastated to have to put my new husband through this and was afraid he would leave. I was perfectly healthy while we were dating and when we got married. "He had not signed up for this," I thought. It was "not part of the plan" according to my "type A" personality.

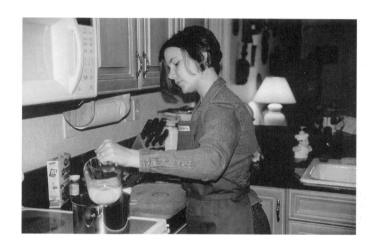

We were relieved when I received the definitive diagnosis three months later; I wasn't dying and I figured I could beat it. I suspected it would be rough later, but that things would be fine until then. Unfortunately, this supposition proved to be wrong time and time again.

Although I came to understand what was going on, it became clear that I was surrounded by two groups of people: those who really "got it" and those who did not. When people do not understand MS, they say things like, "it's not too far to walk," or "it'll be ok, we'll pass a bathroom in twenty minutes." These people certainly don't mean to put you in a bad position, but they can. Perhaps they are in denial that your needs have changed, and will thus end up ignoring them. I have found myself "interviewing" people before spending time with them.

After learning how to deal with these "social" situations, you discover who the valuable people in your life are. My husband did stay with me and has become my number one supporter. He says that he's "not going anywhere," and I'm thankful that I'm not going through this alone. I'm also fortunate to have the tremendous support of my mother and stepfather, Tom.

MS has forced me to change my life plans, to understand who "gets it" and who doesn't, and to appreciate life.

JONATHAN

One of the most common questions I receive, after the obvious, "How's Laural?" is, "…and how are *you* holding up?" I always have, and certainly always will, appreciate when people ask this question. The fact that I'm holding up pretty well seems to have evoked more than a couple of raised eyebrows, so perhaps an explanation is in order.

I don't frighten too easily. That being said, the events surrounding what turned out to be Laural's first exacerbation had me downright petrified. Here we were, married just under a year, twelve thousand-odd miles from home and enjoying a fabulous month-long trip to Australia and New Zealand. When Laural started exhibiting some numbness and stamina problems, my first thoughts were ones of puzzlement: Why was my lovely young bride, some fourteen years my junior, wearing out before I was?

As her mysterious symptoms progressed, we sought the help of a massage therapist, assuming the problem to be one of a pulled muscle or pinched nerve. Obviously, the thought that this problem was a *disease* seemed unthinkable at that point. The therapist agreed that the problem seemed to be something akin to a pinched nerve, and offered Laural some stretching exercises to help work things out—but cautioned that if things didn't improve after a few days, we should seek the advice of a physician.

Several days later, things became much worse, and as we sat in a quaint little hospital in the tiny town of Mossman, Australia, our fears began to grow. The doctor, after doing a handful of standard neurologic tests, was obviously uncomfortable providing us with a diagnosis. She wanted to consult with several colleagues first. She suggested that we return to our hotel, enjoy dinner, and that she'd call us in the morning.

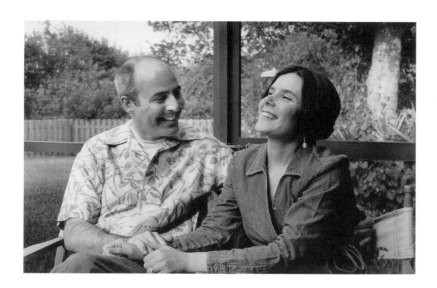

The next morning, the phone rang. It was *the call*. The doctor had spoken with a specialist and they both feared that Laural had either a blood clot on her spine or a very fast-growing cancer pressing up against the spinal cord; either of which would require immediate surgery. In order to better diagnose the situation an MRI was immediately scheduled. In fact, returning to the States wasn't even an option at that point. Until the MRI ruled out something that required surgery, we were stuck.

At the time, I was certainly not sharing my worst fears with Laural, nor was she sharing hers with me. In fact, it wasn't until over a year had gone by that we found out we were both thinking the same thing: Laural wasn't going to make it because it was going to be some sort of inoperable tumor.

When we sat with the doctors a half-hour after she emerged from the machine, and they pointed out her cancer-free, blood clot-free spinal cord, we both cried tears of joy. Yes, there was still something wrong, and yes, we had to leave ten days early, but this was something that could be dealt with. At home.

Thus, my answer. I've dealt with the worst potential news. Yes, MS is a horrible disease; from week to week we don't know what it's going to bring. As frustrating as it is to be socked with physical limitations, we often reflect back on what we thought was going to happen. No, we don't know where MS will take us, but for now, we fight it each and every week with an injection. Even though Laural was trained to self-inject and did so the first couple of times, it makes me feel good that I'm there to do the injections for her.

Her bravery and strength in dealing with this matter have been inspirational. She deserves nothing less that to be married to someone who can "handle" it.

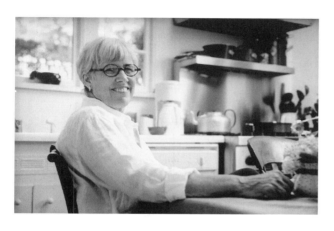

It took me a long time to say, "I have MS." I didn't want to believe it, think it, or live with physical limitations and dependency. In 1995 I was diagnosed, with symptoms having slowly progressed over the preceding years.

My balance is unpredictable, my gait is awkward. I wear a leg brace supported in very ugly shoes. I have diminished stamina and must pace my day carefully.

These things have required enormous changes in daily routine and attitude. Adjustments have come slowly, but on reflecting I am now noticing many positive aspects to these challenges. The need to always be in control has abated. In fact, I'm finding it rather wonderful to accept just letting things be. I am much more open to receiving support and concern. Nurturing myself has become easier and more permissible. I have become more introspective and feel richer emotionally. Priorities are more reasonably aligned; love and gratitude for friends and an incredible family are extremely poignant.

I'm learning to paint. I'm not very good but do enjoy trying and would never have dared before to tap my creative side. Bike rides on our tandem are very much looked forward to. My husband Tom is strong, athletic, attentive and encouraging, and can haul me along behind.

25

There continue to be frustrations, but over all I think I have adapted well and am grateful for what I can do. Awareness that I am much more fortunate than most with this disease is ever apparent.

All sources point to a cure on the horizon.

Please let it be soon!

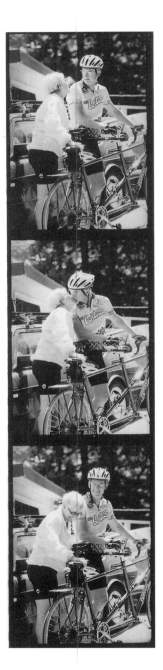

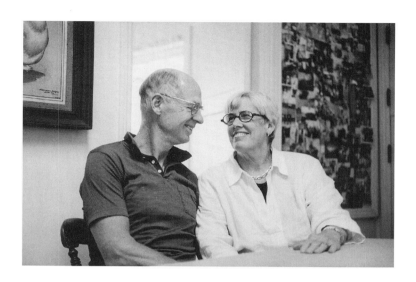

Tom

First, with the realization that my wife, Judy, had multiple sclerosis, came a mixture of painful feelings. Sorrow for her and worry about what the illness would bring led to anger and disappointment knowing that many of the things which we had looked forward to doing together would now be impossible.

Next came a turning away from what had been lost to what was still possible. What had been secondary interests could become more important and new areas could be explored. I began to realize that even with the limitations of illness there was still more to engage in than there was time and energy. Making the most of what we had could be enough.

Still, some regret that this unwelcome illness appeared creeps in from time to time, preventing complete acceptance of our situation and reminding us that life is uncertain.

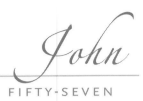

John

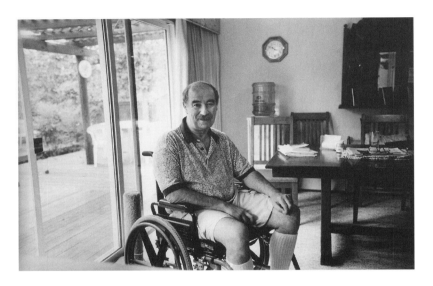

I HAVE NOW HAD MULTI-PLE SCLEROSIS for more than half of my life. I often feel like I have fought all the MS battles there could be. The diagnosis and progressive debilitation have taken me through many changes. As conditions and circumstances change, I somehow adapt. I cannot explain how, but I've done it and know I will keep doing it.

My career was the first to be impacted by circumstances of my diagnosis. After one year in a new job, I had an exacerbation and needed time off. I signed a medical information release form requested by the company. My doctor disclosed a "probable MS" diagnosis to my company doctor, but never let me know, thinking it was "in my best interest" not to tell me. A couple of years later, when complaining to a coworker about my feelings of not being given equal treatment on the job, he said to me, "Go see your doctor." That was how I came to learn I had MS.

I stayed with the company for twenty years, the last four working with real physical limitations, before taking a long-term disability leave. I feel fortunate to have made the best of what could have been a bad situation.

My personal life, especially my marriage, was also rocked. My first marriage lasted several uncomfortable and unhappy years after the diagnosis. The challenge of creeping physical difficulties became too much for both of us. I hated to divorce, especially because of our two children, but believe that she and I are each better off not being together.

While my physical abilities were shifting like loose sand beneath my feet, I needed to keep finding new ways to manage. I somehow weathered the storms emotionally, but the physical toll has been high. I am no longer ambulatory. While there are plenty of things I am unable to do, I concentrate on what I *can* do. And I have been able to maintain a respectable degree of independence. One of the best things for me was to become involved, learning all that I could about MS, and by sharing support with others who have this disease. I am married now to a woman who

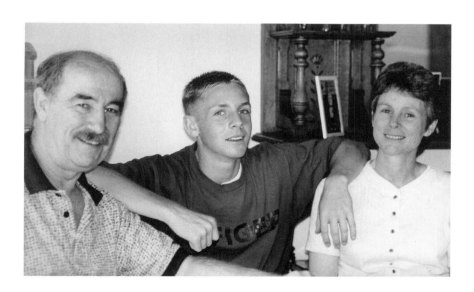

also has MS that I met at a support group. It is a wonderful marriage and we have received enormous rewards raising a great son, Michael.

I do not know what our future holds for us, but I am confident that we will find our way. I do know that I have a wife and three children whom I love deeply, and that everyday I can tell people that, "I am a happy and healthy man who just happens to use a wheelchair."

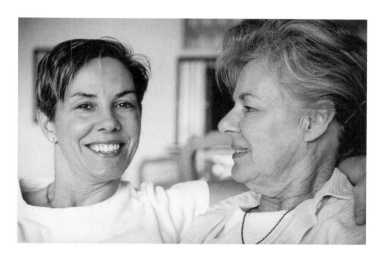

MULTIPLE SCLEROSIS is the Mount Everest of diseases. Just when you think you've reached the summit, you are suddenly faced with decline. Often on the trek, we pass others who have lost the inward struggle and see those who have transformed their lives forever. The challenge of living with MS involves facing ourselves to see who we are as we learn to cope everyday with change. I am an artist, and struggle to discover how I can continue a lifelong pursuit in a new way. MS has forced me to give up my past self and forge ahead with a new identity that accommodates the needs MS has imposed upon me.

I was diagnosed in 1988 with a bilateral vision loss that would last a full year. Like so many others, it came at a time in my life when I was realizing dreams. Barely thirty years old and actively involved in a marketing and advertising career, I was beginning the professional climb of my life. I was also expressing my creative side through a pursuit of photography. The disease would eventually catch up with me, when after a six year remission I was forced to use a wheelchair. That's when I began fighting for my life with everything I have.

MS is a very inconvenient disease that requires a great deal of management and the best tools we can find. You can't climb Mount Everest with an old ice pick. Like anything we do in life, surrounding ourselves with the best equipment, up-to-date information and a good pair of boxing gloves can ensure success in meeting our goals. A better life requires smarter thinking, and a commitment to making a real investment in one's self by taking an honest look at what has changed and what needs to be done to move forward.

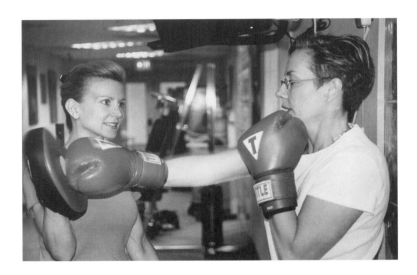

These days, my focus is on MSWorld, an online website I created for people with multiple sclerosis. In creating this site, I've tried to provide the tools to help others begin a new life. Our members include those who are surviving the climb and looking for ways to be better equipped. The website offers freedom from the isolation that accompanies a diagnosis, by giving members a place to connect with others while gathering the latest medical information available. MSWorld is helping thousands every day to reestablish their lives. I've come to realize that most of us are reaching for the best life we can.

Off-line support has been just as vital to my wellness program. I rely heavily on a supportive family and friends to help me out with many day-to-day activities. I work with a massage therapist to help with overall body stiffness and a personal trainer whom I see weekly to help strengthen every muscle that can be strengthened. I believe that these individuals have helped me to realize a healthier physical perspective, which offers me a tremendous amount of hope. I hope to stay well long enough to receive new treatments that might one day cure this disease. Every day I awake with the knowledge that I have a progressive illness and must cope with the possibility that a cure may or may not come about that will halt its progress.

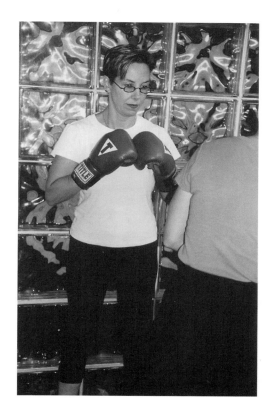

MSWorld reflects the hard-earned wisdom I've gained through the years: *Wellness is a state of mind.* I believe that today is the challenge and tomorrow is the reward. I've come to realize how important it is to take care of myself through exercise, nutrition and positive thinking. And I know now that we can make the most of each day if we're willing to take time to reflect and reach for life's meaning through the chaos. MSWorld is here to facilitate the process of feeling well and to help people discover a better life.

I keep fighting back with the help of others and a digital camera; I am working towards expanding my creative expression once again. The reward comes in the journey and the daily discoveries that I'm making along the way.

33

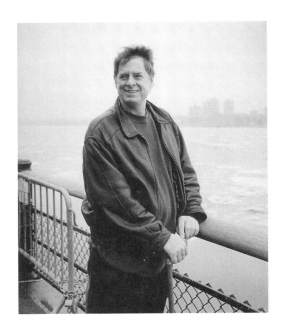

MY CONSTANT COMPANION in life is not my mate, nor my loyal dog. It is my illness, touching everything I do and defining who I am. My gaze into the mirror reveals nothing. Sickness cannot always be seen, but I am ever aware that I am not alone. It is there.

I live with multiple sclerosis, which arrived three decades ago and overstayed its welcome. I cannot get the damned disease out of the house. I have tangoed and tangled, doing battle with MS for my entire adult life. I was a young man when illness arrived, an ambitious television journalist with large hopes for the future. After the bad news came, I was determined to stay the course and build a life. And so I did.

MS and I know each other well. Too well. We are not friends, but "know thy enemy" I always say. MS and I seem to have established an uneasy but calm relationship. Histrionics stormed across the stage long ago. High emotion did not help. I am locked in mortal combat with this predator, and the painful truth is this: the beast will win. As with any disease that is little known and devastating, victory becomes a relative term.

34

My weapon of choice is a strong state of mind, that elusive positive attitude that lets me walk, sometimes hobbling slowly, out of the house each day to do what it is that I do. That is all I can do. My self-confidence stays strong, my determination to succeed unyielding. An arm and leg that no longer function well slow me down. Legal blindness makes the path ahead difficult to see. I am exhausted, and life's little tasks are large obstacles.

But my life is good. Others suffer worse. I will go forward because backward is not acceptable. This is my shot, and the brass ring is out there somewhere. I cannot accept sympathy. I am too busy.

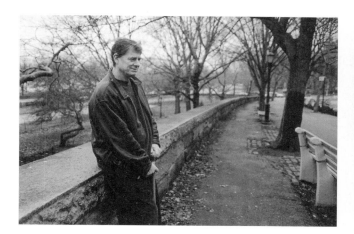

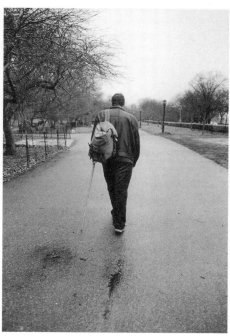

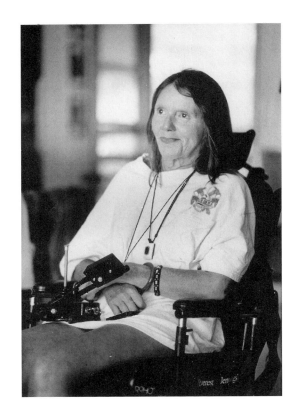

THIS HAS BEEN SUCH an adventure, and it all began fifteen years ago in 1986 when I was diagnosed with MS in September of that year.

Following an initial exacerbation, I had to relearn how to hold a pen and write. I felt overwhelmed when I could no longer function in my workplace nor take care of my animals (one dog, two cats). My boyfriend at that time helped me during his lunch break and after work. However, he was not able to handle the stress surrounding my new situation and soon broke off the relationship.

How did I handle this? I quit my job and began drinking excessively—a habit that became outwardly problematic to me and my loved ones by the end of that year. Drinking quelled my fears but ironically, when I began to face up to it, my MS began to go into remission and I was able to perform some old functions like driving again. There was nothing I could do about the MS but there certainly was something I could do about the drinking. So, early in 1987 I got involved in AA, and I haven't had a drink in fifteen years!

In these past fifteen years I've gone from using a cane, to metal crutches, to a walker, and now to a motorized wheelchair. Earlier in that time period, I started swimming in the bay and using medications to control some of the side effects of this disease. I've never begrudged needing additional assistance but rather have been grateful that such aids have been available.

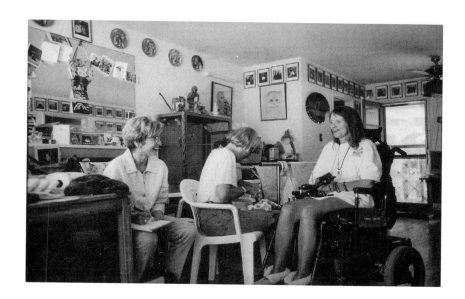

Over the years I've acquired a few more animals including twenty birds, three cats, and now one dog, Goldie, my golden retriever whom I consider my "daughter." I remain in my home alone with the exception of my animals and a caregiver who is here two hours in the morning and one hour in the evening.

I've been buoyed by the tremendous support of a large network of friends and animals. Among my closest friends are over forty firemen who came into my life at a time of great stress. (Five years ago a new man in my life, Bill, learned that he had terminal cancer and the stress of that situation caused a major setback in my MS. Neighbors began to notify the fire department after finding me on the floor of my house and unable to stand.) To show my gratitude for their assistance, I began baking bread using a bread machine. Since then, I've acquired five machines and have provided my "firemen brothers", as well as friends and neighbors, with over 1,500 loaves of bread, earning me the proud e-mail address: "Barbie Bread."

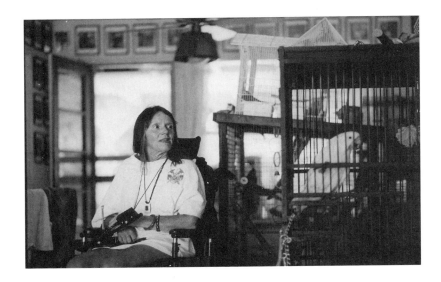

I rarely focus on my obvious situation but rather count the blessings in my life, of which there are many. There are always situations that we as human beings must deal with throughout our lives, and I believe with all my heart that mine is far from the worst. So many people contend with constant pain, both physical and emotional—the knowledge of this provides me with perspective and strength in my life everyday.

Jane

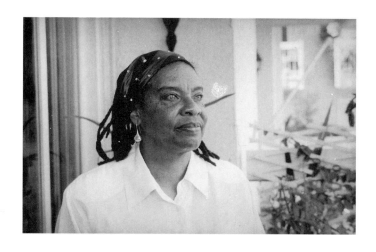

SEPTEMBER 28, 1997 was a very busy day. My husband Guy, some relatives and I would be spending three days on a houseboat. I went to bed that evening very anxious to get away for a few days of relaxation. We were up at 3:00 A.M. the next morning in an attempt to get an early start. As soon as my feet hit the floor, I became aware that my left side was stiff, I was extremely weak, and I was walking with a limp. I was sure after walking a little everything would be just fine. Today I still have stiffness and limp.

After we came home from our short vacation I immediately went to see my chiropractor but got no relief. Next I went to see my general practitioner, who immediately told me she suspected multiple sclerosis. She arranged appointments for me to get an MRI and to see a neurologist.

The neurologist also suspected MS but my MRI did not show enough to indicate a positive diagnosis. The doctor advised me to get as much information as possible about the disease. He advised me to go to the library at Kaiser Hospital, contact the Multiple Sclerosis Society, and to join a support group for the newly diagnosed. Guy and I did all that was suggested and we attended seminars. Friends sent me newspaper articles and I joined a support group, which I learned the most

39

from. It was a pleasure being around others who have the same problems I did and who could provide helpful solutions. Now I belong to two support groups.

Guy is my caregiver and what a blessing! He is very patient with my mood swings. He also has been giving me my weekly injections of interferon for the last two years. My independence is most important. We took yoga classes for over a year. I am in my fourth eight-week session of water aquatics. I now see a naturopathic doctor and have also joined Weight Watchers. I use a cane and own a motorized scooter. I will use anything that will help my mobility or make me feel better. I try to manage my time and activities so that I don't get too exhausted, since fatigue is a major symptom of MS. I work at making my life as normal as possible.

Thanks to Guy, the National MS Society, and my support groups for helping me move forward.

Guy

Editor's Note: *Guy died of cancer in 2002. He will be greatly missed.*

I was injured on my job in May of 1996. I had been working thirty plus years, but had no intentions of retiring. I was being forced into early retirement, something I really had trouble dealing with. I was sitting around the house in a state of depression and feeling sorry for myself.

In October of 1997 Jane got up one morning and said she felt a little stiff. We were on our way to a five-day vacation. We would be spending time on a houseboat on a lake three or four hours away from our home.

Jane thought that the stiffness would pass as she walked around. On the last day of the trip she seemed no better, so upon our return she went to see a doctor. The first thing the doctor said was, "it sounds and looks like multiple sclerosis." Jane had an upper and lower MRI, which showed scarring on her brain.

We tried to learn more about multiple sclerosis. We went to seminars, support groups, the Kaiser Hospital library, and the MS Society. We took yoga, water aerobics, and consulted a naturopathic doctor. Jane and I have learned about MS but are still learning more each day.

I think Jane's attitude and the way she has approached the MS problem has changed the way I look at my own health problems. She has given me strength. I look at things differently now. I try to give Jane my support and I know she does the same for me. We've grown closer, and we try to enjoy every moment.

Jane was a go-getter person before MS. Now, she has to take things a little slower and is in the house more than she wants to be. We still try to get out as much as possible, and we try to laugh as much as we can.

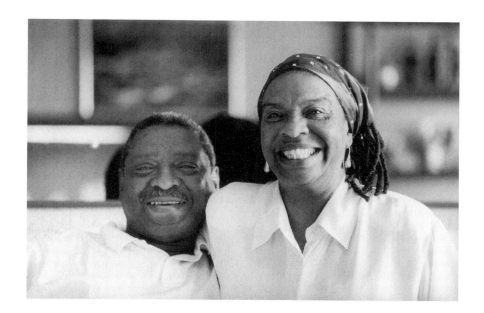

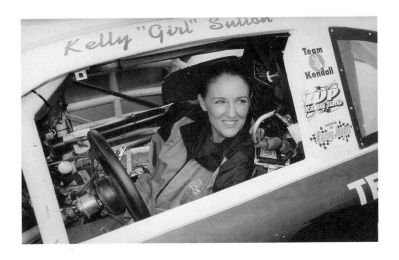

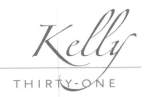

To some, growing up in the arena of racing may seem quite strange and unimaginable. But for our family, working on the racecar through the weekdays and traveling to local racetracks on the weekends was as natural as having meals together. Watching my father win races and marveling at his competitive spirit reinforced one thought, I wanted to be just like him. At five years old, I choose my profession—I wanted to be a racecar driver.

I was a tomboy at heart with a competitive personality. Some of my friends had tea parties and played with paper dolls. I played softball, rode bicycles, mini bikes, motorcycles, and raced go-carts. Advancing in these sports seemed like a natural progression for me. After all, I was focused on my ultimate dream, to race at Daytona—someday.

It was obvious by the age of thirteen that something was happening to me. I was no longer the fastest runner on my ball team; I was clumsy, and tired most all of the time. I thought that if I slept enough, I would feel better. My mom thought we should see a doctor. That marked the beginning of a three-year journey that included diagnoses from viruses, "just adolescence," to

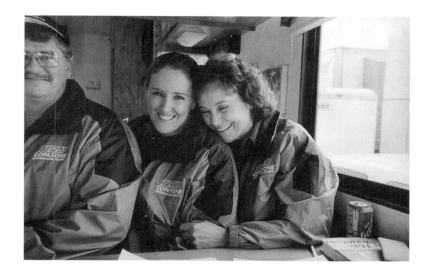

depression—not to mention hypochondria. Any pain that I was feeling "was just in my head."

We continued on this same path until one night the right side of my body became numb. Mom's intuition and persistence won, and we were finally referred to a neurologist. Soon I underwent a series of tests that would confirm I had multiple sclerosis. I didn't know what MS was; but I did know it wasn't "in my head."

At sixteen we plan to get our driver's license, attend proms and homecomings, and prepare for graduation. I had also planned to enter my first racecar competition. Instead, I was tutored my final five months of high school. Through the help of a tutor in high school, I did get to walk across the graduation stage; however, I did not get to race. To me, MS would rob me of every challenge life could offer—sentencing me to a wheelchair for life.

The journey between diagnosis and where I am today had many detours. Disbelief and denial were my initial reactions, keeping my feelings hidden from even my best friend. My competitive spirit was gone and I was angry. A deep black hole of depression encompassed my soul. I might have stayed in this place had I not been blessed with a family that believed in me and convinced me to believe in myself.

I started educating myself about MS. Understanding the disease gave me the power to direct my life and revisit my childhood dream of being a racecar driver. I accepted that I had MS—MS didn't have me. In time, therapies became available and I searched until I found the one that worked for me. And—I am pursuing my dreams. I am a racecar driver, and yes, I have raced on the high banks of Daytona International Speedway. I compete on the racetrack to win! I compete with MS to win as well! Sharing the knowledge with others that life does not end after diagnosis is my victory of fifteen years ago, when MS took control of my life. Today, with a positive attitude, supportive family, friends, and managed health care (including exercise and diet), I am in the driver's seat.

As you run your race with MS, I'd like to share some things that I have learned. *Do* seek early therapy, it could make the difference; *do* reach out to other people, they will give you strength. *Do* continue to believe in yourself and have dreams—dreams really can come true. And, I have only one "don't," *don't* give up, that is the only thing that will limit you.

CAROL

"Mrs. Sutton, line two." It was a cold winter day in February when I received the call.

A mother's intuition is generally accurate; so it was with mine. Desperate to find an answer, I had taken my daughter, Kelly, from doctor to doctor only to receive a myriad of diagnoses. Something not yet identified was lurking in my child's body—not "in her mind" as emphatically told to me by one medical professional. I knew there was a reason why Kelly felt pain, that she slept more than a normal young girl did, and that her gait was off. Now, nearly four years later, the mystery was solved—Kelly's disease had been identified.

"Hello, this is Carol Sutton." My heart sank as I heard the voice of the neurologist I had taken Kelly to see earlier in the week. He spoke without emotion and to the point, "…Kelly's test results indicate… she has multiple sclerosis. I'd like to send her for a spinal tap and to Johns Hopkins for a second opinion."

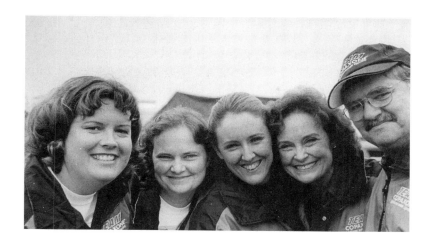

Although surrounded by coworkers, I felt totally alone at that moment. The instinctive feeling that had kept me searching for an answer was suddenly replaced with shock and fear. *"God, no, please no, not Kelly, please take this from her. Give it to me—take me—she is so young. Dear God, I beg you, please!"* Sobbing so hard I could not speak, my boss sent me home from work. How was I going to tell my daughter—and our family?

I knew nothing of the disease; only that a woman from our church had recently died from complications of MS. *"No! I can't think that now; I must be positive!"* Kelly could not know that I was scared beyond words. A mother shields and protects her children from harm, soothes and comforts them when they are ill. Yet, all the nurturing I had to give could never take this disease away. I felt so helpless.

The agony of looking into my beautiful daughter's big brown eyes and seeing her countenance of terror is still indelible in my mind. The neurologist at John Hopkins told Kelly she should not have children; it could exacerbate the disease. Perhaps she would have eight to ten years before using a wheelchair. I tried to bargain with God, *"please take my life Lord, give it to Kelly."* I am grounded in my faith enough to know we don't bargain with God, but in that moment of despair, hope seemed far from view.

45

Kelly progressively got worse. My husband carried her to the bathroom, she stopped eating and slept most of the time. I truly thought Kelly was dying. The future held multiple episodes of relapse after relapse followed by a time of abatement. We learned that Kelly's type of MS was relapsing/remitting.

As a caregiver, I silently carried my fears and talked to God often. I was tired, both mentally and physically, but never abandoned the desire to make life better for Kelly. I worked hard at encouraging her to never give up—trusting and believing that she could overcome life's obstacles. I searched for resources that would educate us about MS.

Fifteen years later, Kelly is effectively managing her disease. Indulging in self-pity is not her style. She has a daughter, is still walking, racing stockcars, and has been blessed with the opportunity to touch the lives of others living with MS. Kelly's strong will and tenacity is an inspiration to me.

Facing our life-changing experiences has been undoubtedly difficult. Although we can manage the disease for now, predicting the future is not ours. Therefore, I choose to control my mind with positive thoughts. I've learned to count each moment a blessing. Our faith keeps us focused, our determination keeps us challenged, and we begin each day with confident expectation that a cure is very close.

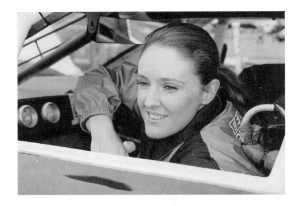

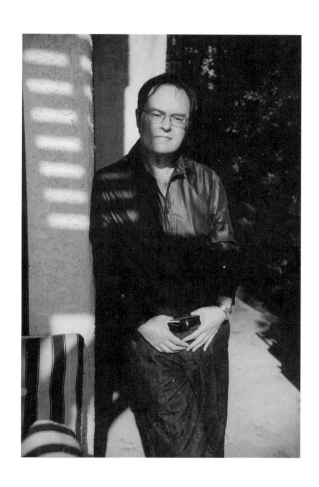

WHEN I WAS INITIALLY DIAGNOSED, the doctor told me I'd never walk again. That was in 1984 when the only way MS could be treated was with mega-doses of prednisone (steroids). Well, after two days of megadosing, I walked out of the hospital determined never to tell anyone what I had. And for fifteen years I kept it a secret, shared only with my wife and daughter. If word got out, I figured nobody would hire me for acting roles. With MS there are so many things that can go wrong: your legs, your eyes, your memory, your speech. . . well you don't need any of that stuff to act, do 'ya?

So for fifteen years we kept it secret which I don't mind saying was a lonely experience. When things went wrong who could I tell? Four years ago I broke my silence and came out of the closet. Since then I've spoken to thousands like myself with this disease and discovered it's great to see that I'm not alone. One of the first

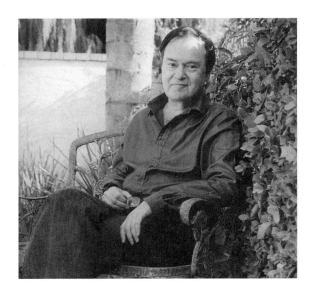

letters I got after *People* magazine announced I was hiding MS read, "Dear Dave, Glad you went public. I've had MS for twenty years. Welcome to the club."

I guess it is a club, though not one I wanted to join voluntarily, but now that I'm in it and I've met the members, I'm proud to include myself.

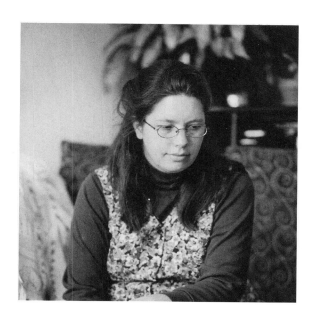

Having MS and being a mother is hard. Because I never know what will affect me, or how my MS will turn out, it is kind of a gamble. Naturally I want to win that gamble. Some people may think it is selfish to want to have kids in spite of this illness, but for me it would be far more selfish not to have children because they force me to consider my ailments in light of their own needs, and in turn I am more connected to the world through them. No space for self-pity there.

The things I cannot provide for them physically I must be clever about. I must use reason instead of force to raise them. They (including the unborn one as well), get a lot of support through friends, neighbors, and family. I nurture the relationships around me a great deal, and people have come to our aid in times of need. I am sad at times to see the things I cannot do for them, but then everyone has limitations and I am always mindful of the fact that kids are very adaptable and helpful—at least most of the time! My husband is the main reason that I decided to go ahead and have children (I once thought I wouldn't), and he has been all the things I cannot be. Although

49

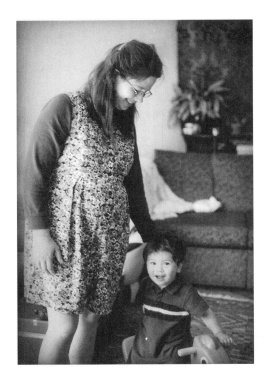

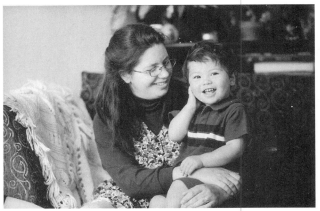

they are a lot of work, I consider our kids to be his greatest gift to me, because without him I never would have thought myself capable of being a mother.

When I lived alone with MS, I was bound and determined to be self-sufficient—to the point of self-destructiveness, but now that I am part of a family, I feel that I am part of a larger community and that even though it is hard, I can ask for help.

Having children has helped give me a direct connection to the "outside" world, from which I may have otherwise cut myself off from because of my illness.

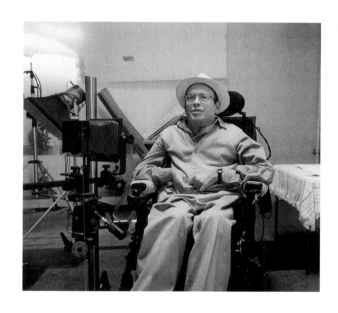

"No one escapes being burned." "If I don't do this, I'm going to be toast!" We all want to avoid the horrific experience of going up in smoke, but not one of us ever does. There are various degrees of burn, but no one is immune. If we look at a variety of bread available today, we could find a metaphor for all humanity. Toast can represent all races and nationalities—and their common suffering. The whitest toast can be burnt black. The dry toast of dieters brings to mind deprivation. French toast may be a symbol of decadence. Toast golden and perfectly done—warm, fragrant and comforting, can be a symbol of perfection as well as destruction.

Likewise, life is not entirely tragic. There are good things: Reggie Jackson's home runs in the World Series, anything by Miles Davis, Woody Allen movies, and the look on a beautiful woman's face when you kiss her for the first time. But the next tragedy is inevitable, no matter how you try to avoid it. Sometimes we jump in the toaster all by ourselves.

Living and working with MS has made my life difficult, but I have to work—it is the most important thing there is. When I work I figure out what I want to do then find the means to get to the point where I can accomplish what I preconceived in my mind. So work hard at whatever you do and the rewards and benefits will overwhelm you. A disabled person should always stand on his/her work as opposed to having someone look at their disability and say, "what they did is good for a disabled person." Being disabled is tough, but it's worse if someone feels sorry for you.

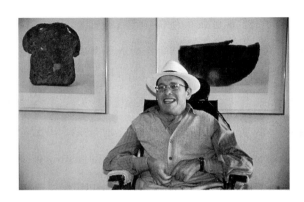 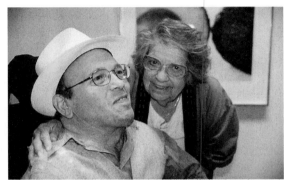

Yes, I have multiple sclerosis, but it is not what defines me. I will never embrace this disease. I will never give it credit for what I have accomplished, and I will never use it as an excuse for what I didn't do. It is something I live with every day, something that influences my experiences and decisions, but not something I wholeheartedly accept. Some may argue that this is not a healthy perspective, but I disagree. To me, MS is a potential limitation, and I refuse to accept any limitations in my life. I will make allowances for my disease, there are things it has already taken from me, but I am not going to surrender. I will live my life with multiple sclerosis, but multiple sclerosis will never be my life.

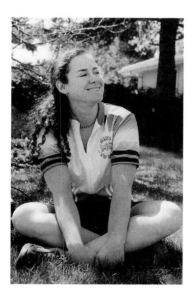 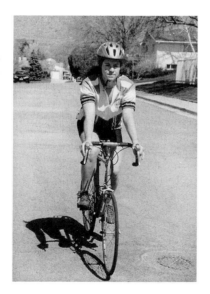

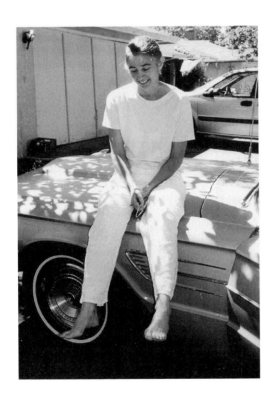

I WISH MS had not surprised me, had not stolen my dreams so quickly. I wonder how my children will remember me. Will they think back on how we challenged the world together or will they be overwhelmed with how our lives have changed?

I hope people remember that when MS first came careening into our lives I had the sense to reach out to a close circle of friends for support and companionship. I organized monthly gatherings at my home, and we shared potluck lunches, recipes, and the warmth of each others' stories. These meetings changed my perspective on the world, strengthened my kids, and offered my friends a glimpse of how one copes with a chronic disease.

Last year I moved to the country and monthly lunches evolved into weekly group e-mails. Oh, the glories of the internet! Seated at my computer every Monday morning I still feel as if my friends are sitting next to me as I regale them with images and observations of small town life in the mountains of northern California. They plan to visit this fall; mostly to see for themselves whether or not I am telling the truth about the beauty and serenity of this place.

My friends watched me learn to be calm and patient as my world changed from a place of risk and discovery to one fashioned by unexpected limitations. It takes a certain brand of courage to survive the uncertainty that is MS. I hope a cure will be discovered. I would love another chance to serve an ace or walk in the rain. Another chance to feel the many rhythms of the day.

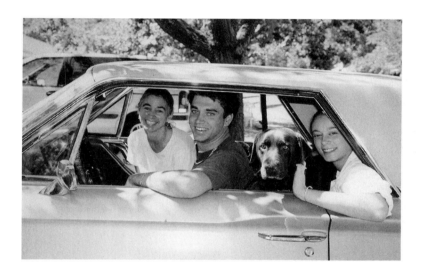

TOMMY

When I was a kid I thought my mom was invincible. I was sure she was going to live forever, that nothing would ever slow her down. Then she got multiple sclerosis. I didn't know what MS was at first, I just knew it was bad because she seemed afraid and I had never seen her frightened of anything before. She told me and my sister that everything was all right and that she would be o.k., but she never let on as to how bad the disease could become.

As I got older I learned more about the course of the disease and how it affects people differently, and I began to realize what frightened my mom. She had been an athlete all her life, playing Division I sports all through college and then coaching me and Rachel when we were young.

Mom loved hiking through the woods and taking long walks along the beach but now, with each passing day, she had to watch her strength and coordination slowly disappear. I think that if anything could have happened to my mom this was the worst because it took away many of the things she loved.

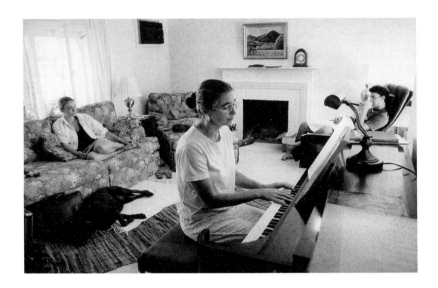

Yet what does not disappear and will never ever go away is the twinkle in her eye and her absolute zest for life. She gets more out of life than anyone I have ever been around, whether she is singing one of her random songs or working on a crossword puzzle. She is quick to laugh and always ready to help the people she loves. She may no longer be invincible but I know her spirit is immortal and it will always live in me.

RACHEL

When I wrote an application essay to get into Princeton, I talked about the moment I'd been hit with the seriousness of my mother's disease; a moment, "when I realized my mother was all too mortal."Those words may have helped me get into college but as I look back upon them, now four years older and wiser, I could not have been more mistaken.

What I'd thought was "mortality" I know now was and is the sign of an unsinkable personality. My mother has not lost any of the intelligence, elegance or incurable optimism that she exhibited before being diagnosed. If anything, it is only more evident now. In the face of something terrible, something that threatened to take away the most cherished aspects of her life, in the immortal words of William Ernest Henley, "in the fell clutch of circumstance" she has not "winced or cried aloud."

She is the epitome of an unconquerable spirit, and she remains the standard to which I can only hope to compare myself. She continues to enchant everyone she comes in contact with. Her laughter is contagious and eternal, and she never ceases to amaze me with her ability to make light of any situation. She is my sun, my moon, and all my stars!

I WAS TWENTY YEARS OLD and considered to be in the prime of my life. I was in college. I had a serious girlfriend with whom I was spending the summer in my hometown of Avalon on Santa Catalina Island, California. I was looking forward to a fun filled summer.

During the previous year I had had several incidents of weakness in my legs, as well as blurred vision, extreme fatigue, and occasional difficulty talking. I was attributing all of these strange happenings to my schoolwork and responsibilities, partying, and just being twenty! My aunt and uncle were the doctors at the hospital in Avalon. My uncle was the surgeon and GP and my aunt the pediatrician and anesthesiologist. Both of them noticed my strange gait and the fact that I would bump into them when we walked together. After several discussions with my parents and local friends my aunt and uncle asked me to come in for an examination. After several examinations and frank discussions it was decided that I should go back to Los Angeles to White Memorial Hospital for further neurologic tests and spinal taps.

After a battery of the same I was diagnosed with multiple sclerosis. I was then informed that no one had knowledge of the cause or cure of this disease. I carried on for several years with standard medical procedures, including steroids and blood thinners. As nothing seemed to be bringing about any changes in the condition I finally decided to take charge of my own case. I reduced my stress load, changed my diet, reduced my dependence on medicines and drug therapies, and began to investigate alternative methods of treatment.

I put my college education on hold and devoted my time and energy to helping myself come to terms with this diagnosis. The promising results of my investigation proved to me that I was on the right track. I just knew I had to find a system that I could incorporate into my life in order to stay in touch with my goals and remain an effective and contributing member of my community.

One of the most intriguing parts of my investigation was hatha yoga. I began studying all the books I could find on the subject. I also began talking with practitioners of yoga and looking for

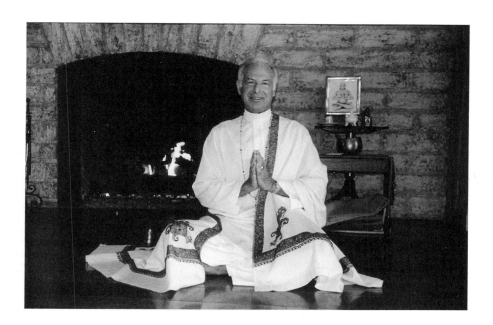

instructors who could help me improve my situation. It wasn't easy. I began studying with Indra Devi, the greatest female instructor of the twentieth century. Through her compassion, knowledge and plain good spirits she pointed me in the right direction and suggested that I also make contact with Satchitananda, a renowned teacher of Integral Yoga who, at the time, was teaching in Santa Barbara. I soon experienced not only an improvement in my health but also a marked improvement in my ability to deal with MS.

I then began to hear about BKS Iyengar and his work in the therapeutic application of hatha yoga with students with various medical conditions. There were many other yoga teachers that I experienced over the years but it was BKS Iyengar's work that proved to be the most effective for me. I was so excited with the results of my studies and practice with Mr. Iyengar that I devoted all my time and energy to his teachings. With each passing day I improved not only physically, but psychologically, spiritually and emotionally. Mr. Iyengar's advice to me after several years of study was that I should teach others like myself.

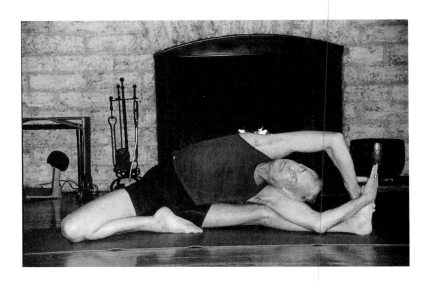

I went back to college, completed my studies with a masters degree in fine arts, obtained a teaching certificate from the state of California, and, while holding down a successful full-time career as a fine arts teachers in the California public schools, obtained a teaching certificate from Mr. Iyengar. Soon after this I began my career teaching therapeutic Iyengar yoga to other people who had been diagnosed with multiple sclerosis. I later married, had three children, and competed successfully as an amateur horse owner in the equestrian arena. That covers the last forty years of turning a negative into a positive!

There now exists the very successful Eric Small Adaptive Yoga Program with the MS Society of California. I have traveled nationally and internationally, conducting workshops for MS clients and hatha yoga teachers. I am the proud grandfather of two of the most adorable grandchildren one could possibly imagine and am very proud of my daughter and son that they also contribute to the welfare and well being of those around them and their community. MS is not the end, it is only the beginning of knowing your full potential. The diagnosis of MS is the opportunity to bring those positive elements that each one of us has and to use them in service of our fellow man.

EDEN

Growing up, my dad was different from the dads of my school friends. I can say this now, looking back on my life. At the time, he was just my dad. I don't really remember knowing that he had MS or what that really meant. He wasn't the type of father who played sports or watched them for that matter. He did ride and compete as an equestrian, and was quite good as I remember, for there were a lot of ribbons hung up on the wall from various competitions.

MS is a disease that affects your nervous system, so we never went anywhere on vacation that was too "cold." He always said that cold weather didn't make him feel well, so we went on beach vacations, Hawaii, Catalina Island, etc., never skiing!!

I remember one specific time when he was very sick and in bed for a few weeks at home—maybe I was 10 or 11—he had a hard time standing up and lost his balance quite a bit. It was around that time, I suppose, that he took up yoga. He turned his office into a studio with huge mirrors and equipment. He began to wear Indian curtas and beads and his balance did improve— I don't remember him being sick again.

The yoga definitely changed his life and now others are being changed now as well. He is very inspirational to me as a teacher-sharing what he went through to help others now afflicted with MS. He looks much younger than his years and it is because of his devotion to yoga. I am so proud to be his daughter!!

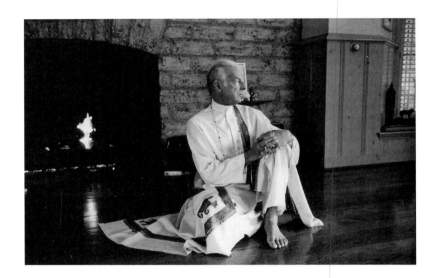

TREVOR

It is an interesting question to ponder; what is it like to grow up with a parent who has the diagnosis of multiple sclerosis. I am not sure of when I exactly became aware that something was different about my father. I had assumed that all fathers needed to take a nap each day. I had assumed a great many things about the way things should be until maybe I was about six. I do recall wanting to play baseball with my father. I had a mitt, ball, and hat and was ready. We stood at opposite ends of the grass and he said, "go ahead, throw it." I threw the ball with the excitement of a six year-old. It flew over his head. He said, "I can't get it, please go get it." I saw then that things were different from what I had seen on television. I saw in his eyes that he wasn't able to do the things that he wanted to with his son. But, and this is a very important but, he would try. My dad was the kind of father who would try something with me and then, at a certain point, I could tell that he couldn't go anymore. That his body just wouldn't do what he wanted it to do.

As a child, I found myself tailoring experiences and activities so that they would be manageable. For example, my father would take my sister and I roller-skating. It was very comical; this tall, thin man scooting around on wheels. After a while, it would be just my sister and I with my father napping on the grass or giving encouragement from the sidelines. I imagine that my father had to really push himself when I was a child and it was hard, I think, to completely understand this. As a kid, I think that I often took my father's fatigue or frustration as having to do with raising me as opposed to the struggles and trials he was dealing with. Sometimes, I wish that I would have known what he was really up against when I was growing up.

From a father's point of view now, I believe that my own father must have been quite frustrated about not being able to run, jump, wrestle, and play all the time. I see now that as a grandfather, he is so energized and excited to play with my son that he will push himself to the point of absolute fatigue just to push the swing one more time. My father has not let multiple sclerosis keep him from life. From the people that I have met with whom he has contact with and teaches, I understand that he is a motivating guide. Sometimes it is easier to just sit down and stop fighting but that is not something that I have ever seen from my father.

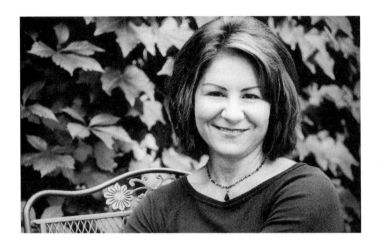

I WAS LIVING THE PICTURE PER-FECT LIFE with three healthy children—Melissa, Todd, and Michael, a loving husband named Steve, and owned a successful business. Then, on July 12, 1991, the day I was diagnosed with multiple sclerosis, I felt my entire world collapse around me. Suddenly, I was immobile—forced to rely on a motorized scooter to get around, and suffering from fatigue. I became withdrawn and depressed.

I kept asking, "Why me?" I thought perhaps I was being punished for having such a wonderful life. I spent my days feeling sorry for myself, mourning the loss of my old life—a life filled with family activities, athletics, and an active social life.

Knowing there was no cure for MS, I tried every treatment possible to beat this disease. After trying diets and herbs—even traveling to Israel to participate in a trial drug study to no avail, I became an angry, bitter and sad person. My family and friends could only hope that I would come to accept my new life with MS—a journey they were willing to help me take. Bless them for their patience.

I reached a turning point after seeing the movie *Schindler's List* with a close friend. Inspired and touched by the story, I realized what I had been doing wrong. Watching the courage of Oskar Schindler save over a thousand lives with the help of those who were suffering in the concentration camps, I had a breakthrough moment. I realized that true peace of mind was not about whether my legs worked or whether I could get my old life back. True survival was survival of my spirit, my attitude—no matter what. And I had been killing my spirit. Suddenly, my pity party ended.

When my attitude changed, everything changed at home. Laughter, music and joy filled our home, our children brought their friends over again, and Steve and I began to discover new ways to enjoy life.

Since my passion is youth, I began to volunteer at Our Friends' Place, a safe haven for abused girls in Dallas, and to speak with teens at the Dallas Memorial Center for Holocaust Studies. The more service work I did with teens, the better I felt. The disease didn't go away; I still suffered fatigue and weakness in my legs, but I began to heal the sadness, fear and anger I had lived with for so long.

Eager to share the power of giving, I decided to compile a book of true stories to inspire others to have the courage to give. My first book, *The Courage to Give*, depicts thirty stories of people who have had something happen to them physically and/or emotionally, whose lives changed miraculously when they started helping others. I now have completed five books as a part of *The Courage to Give* series, with over a hundred courageous people confirming the power of giving.

I travel across the country speaking to people with MS. Hopefully, they will all discover the unique gifts we are all given to share with others. I encourage others with MS to find the courage to give—to put aside the challenges of the disease and reach out to help someone else—with the hope that they, too, will discover what I continue to learn; that when we help others, we begin to feel better physically and spiritually.

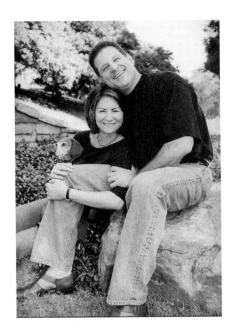

Our caregivers—family, friends, and great doctors—are a blessing in our lives. We cherish their help, support, and love. But, no one can fix our attitude for us. To choose to live life to its fullest, no matter what, begins within each of us.

I believe having MS has been a blessing. Through helping others I continue to learn important life lessons. Our family is closer than ever; we laugh and love our life. We don't "sweat the small stuff." With their help and my change of heart, I have been able to learn the joy of giving and receiving.

Living with MS is a challenge. But, true survival is survival of our spirit, no matter what. Our loved ones don't care if we can't do what we used to do; they just want us to be who we used to be. There is always someone worse off than we are. It's our responsibility while we live on this planet to remember who we really are—souls filled with love and the desire to give. When we choose to remember and take action to help others, our MS becomes only a part of who we are, and our lives become bigger, richer, and perhaps better than ever.

STEVE

I will always remember the first time I met Jackie. I was fifteen; we were at a youth dance. I saw this gorgeous girl in a pink dress sitting in a chair across the room. Her perfect posture, captivating smile, and sparkling eyes intrigued me. They still do.

Our marriage of thirty one years has been a journey filled with joy, sadness, love and discovery. When Jackie was initially diagnosed with MS, I told her we would get through this together. I knew I could handle this—that's my nature. Little did I know how MS would affect our lives; how it would take much more than the conviction that our lives could remain the same and all would be fine.

Watching my soul mate face the challenges of living with MS has changed me as well as her. It's difficult to watch someone we love struggle. As a husband, best friend and lover, I wanted for so long to make her as happy and comfortable as possible. It has taken both of us a long time to come to terms with the realities of the disease.

Adapting to a slower lifestyle, making sure Jackie got enough rest, and balancing the symptoms with trying to make life "normal" with our children and our marriage, all proved to be more than I ever imagined. And the girl I fell in love with was lost, buried in self-doubt, sadness and physical pain. I wanted so badly to make things better. I wanted to fix this problem. But I couldn't.

I kept remembering the girl I married—the girl with spunk, drive, and a loving nature. I had faith that one day she would find that person again and we would all be fine.

Thank God that day arrived. When Jackie chose to change her attitude, our lives did change. And our marriage is stronger than ever. We take joy in the little things; we do things differently, but that's okay. And, best of all, we are caregivers for each other, knowing that in the giving we receive.

There have been difficult moments and I know there will be more. But with or without MS, that girl I first saw over thirty-five years ago is back—and I'm forever grateful.

MELISSA

I wondered why my mom took a nap every afternoon. But, I never thought twice about how my friends and I would hang out in my parents' room after school—because that's where my mom would be, in bed. It wasn't until I was seventeen that it all made sense. My mom was diagnosed in 1991 with multiple sclerosis, and severe fatigue was one of her symptoms.

At first, the diagnosis was frightening. Our family didn't know what that meant and of course I thought the worst. Restricted to a motorized scooter, my mom was devastated.

Finally, mom decided she wasn't going to let MS take away her life. Although she had fatigue, she began volunteering in the community. And the service she did for others gave her new energy and a new perspective. She discovered that although she couldn't find the cure for MS, she could find joy and love.

My mom decided to write a book, *The Courage to Give*, which contains inspiring stories of people who have encountered tragedy in their lives and made the best of it. She has now written three other books and has been able to share her story and the courageous stories of others with America. Through her example, my mom has taught me (along with millions of others) the most important lesson I have learned in life—faced with any challenge, if we serve others, miraculously, we can begin to heal.

I got married last year and both my mom and dad walked me down the aisle.

MICHAEL

I was eleven years old and had just returned from summer camp when I found out my mother had multiple sclerosis. My memory of that day is a mixture of what I actually remember, and what has been told to me over the years. My older brother and I were in the car riding home from the airport when we were told. The first question that popped into our heads was answered before we had even posed the question: "This disease is not fatal, I will not die from it." These words from

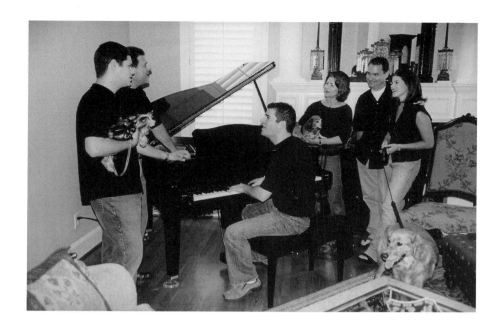

my mother were comforting. In my mind (knowing nothing about the disease and being too young to comprehend the severity of such an illness), this was not a big deal. So my mom had a disease. It couldn't kill her, so what was the big deal?

In later years, as I grew older, I gained a better understanding of MS. The disease itself was a much bigger deal than I had originally thought. The neurologic and emotional effects of the disease could in fact severely affect a patient's normal way of life. My mother, however, never let that happen. Her positive outlook on life and her situation made it seem as if nothing was wrong.

My experience growing up with a mother who had MS was like any other kid, with three exceptions. My mom tired more than other moms, which required her to rest more; she had back pain, which required a nightly ritual of "Push Right Here"—now known in our family as "PRH," and occasionally, there was a little mood swing from time to time (I tried to stay out of the way as much as possible!).

Besides these small things, my mother's outlook on everything really laid the path for the rest of us to follow. We all pitched in, we all helped out, and we were still the same loving family that every other family dreams of, but may not get to experience. Even though my mother has MS, my family considers themselves privileged to be around someone who is such a caring and kind person to everyone she encounters, and who has accomplished more in half of her lifetime than most people can in two.

TODD

Upon our arrival at the airport, my brother Michael and I were met by our parents. We had just spent several months away at summer camp and were elated to return home to the comfort of our family. My father opened his arms and warmly embraced us as we disembarked; however, my mother's response was quite different. Sitting by herself in the corner of the baggage-claim area, her body language did not match the welcoming temperament of my father, but was unusually cold, reflective and isolated. Initially, anger brewed inside of me. I was irritated that my own mother was too selfish to be happy to see her son after two months; after all, I was merely fourteen. Subsequently, as rational feelings took hold I started to question *why* she was not her natural self. As we drove home from the airport, I deduced that there was some kind of serious predicament. Finally, I just blurted out, "What is mom's problem?" To which my father responded after glancing sympathetically at my mother, "We have something to tell you."

The news was horrible and yet hazy at the same time since my brother and I really did not really understand. What was multiple sclerosis? Was there a cure? Was mom going to die? I may not have fully grasped the details of the disease, but my mother's expressions were unbearable; I just wanted so badly for her to be her happy, outgoing self again.

As much as I wanted and tried to help, giving her foot and back massages to increase her circulation or making hilarious jokes at dinner to try and lighten up the mood, her self-confidence and zest for life had simply vanished. Sure, we all adapted to the situation, but my father was amazing to us, truly vital in dispelling our frustration with her incessant sadness. The hardest part of those few years for me was that I loved my mother so much, but was just so angry at her for being upset. She had always told me that life is what you make of it and accordingly, any goal was within my reach as long as I worked hard and desired to succeed. If she practiced what she preached, then why couldn't my mother just snap out of it? Didn't she *want* to feel better? It took me a while, but my father helped me accept the fact that, during that difficult time, mom just wasn't herself.

Since then, so much has changed for the better, and my mother has truly become an inspiration for all of us. She proved to me and everyone else that life *is* what you make of it. No matter what happens, life does not revolve around the self, but the self revolves around life!

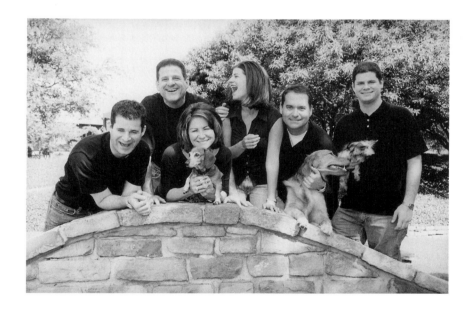

Consider it pure joy, my brothers, whenever you face trials of many kinds,

because you know that the testing of your faith develops perseverance.

Perseverance must finish its work so that you may be mature and complete,

not lacking anything. James 1:2-4

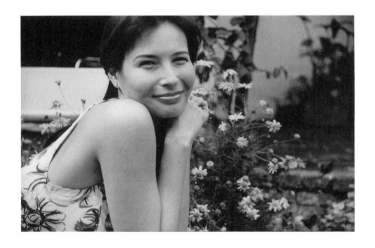

DREAMS. They are always lingering in the depths of your subconscious, sneaking up on you when you least expect it. I think that I was three years old when I decided I wanted to be Miss America. And then I really didn't think about it until my senior year in high school when my college counselor told me I was running in Hawaii's Junior Miss contest. My background made me the perfect candidate; I was a nerd who had not only won a grand prize in Microbiology at the State Science Fair, but top place at a national dance competition with Drill Team Hawaii. I was also on the student council, the swim and tennis teams, had performed in every school play and musical, and volunteered as a Big Sister, a tutor, and treasurer of the EARTH Club. I needed the scholarship money and I loved performing onstage, so I said ok. To my surprise I won the Fitness, Presence and Composure, and Top

Scholar awards. And that is how the girl who never wore makeup ended up representing Hawaii at America's Miss Junior Miss Pageant.

While pageants are sometimes considered shallow spectacles that are demeaning to women, my experience was empowering. Having a voice in the community that was amplified by a title was an awesome honor and a responsibility I enjoyed. The dream had resurfaced, and when I graduated from Yale University it finally refused to be ignored.

January 13, 2001 was one of the happiest days of my life. I had just been crowned Miss Waikiki, and I was looking forward to competing at Miss Hawaii. No matter the outcome I felt my dream had come true. I would have the opportunity to showcase my talent singing on television and win scholarships to help pay off the massive loans my father took out to send me to college. That night was full of excitement and possibilities. I felt wonderful, but then I noticed a different sensation; my feet and legs felt numb and tingly.

At first I just thought it was my big 'ol, Hawaiian feet rebelling against my four-inch pageant heels. But the strange sensations didn't go away and over the course of a month they enveloped my torso and spread out to my hands. After seeking medical help, my neurologist immediately checked me into the hospital. He thought I might have a tumor on my spine, a scary thought which I didn't believe for a moment. What I wasn't told was that he really suspected worse—a rapidly metastasizing brain cancer. After five days of tests, including blood work, x-rays, a spinal tap, and MRIs of my brain and spine, I was told I had multiple sclerosis.

I felt relieved. I was right, no tumor. And then I realized I was puzzled because I didn't have a clue as to what MS was, even though I had volunteered at a MS fundraiser in high school.

But this is a marvelous age for accessible information, so filling the gap in my knowledge of MS came easily. My wonderful family and friends not only rallied around me with love and emotional support, but showered me with books, pamphlets and videos about MS; you name it, I probably have it. I also searched the internet and found numerous helpful websites and, after a call to the

National MS Society, a huge packet of information arrived in the mail. I was empowering myself with knowledge.

However, as I learned more about MS I had to decide that I would not live in fear. It is frightening indeed to learn that there are so many unknowns in the realm of MS and that there is still no cure. I began to feel all my dreams slip out of the reach of my numb hands. Would I be able to compete at Miss Hawaii? Would I ever be on Broadway or in a movie? Would I get married and have a family? Would I still change the world? The questions were interrupted by a visit from my

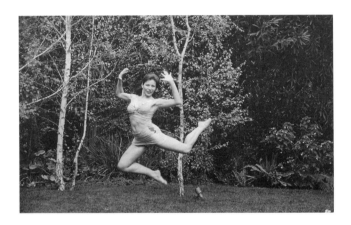

pastor who gave me life-changing and inspiring advice. Pastor Wayne encouraged me not to ask, "Why God? Why me? Why now?" but to ask, "What is your plan, Lord? How can I use this to help others?" He helped me to realize that the only thing that would keep me from reaching my dreams was *me*. I left the hospital with the decision that in my small way I would join the fight against MS, assist in raising awareness and funds for research and a cure, and help others who suffer from this devastating disease in any way I could. Personal education was not enough. Action was called for!

In July 2002 my perseverance paid off. After fracturing my back in a horseback riding accident I decided to enter another pageant to give myself a goal for my recovery. Five weeks later I became

America's first Miss Intercontinental. Winning a national pageant has given me a priceless and powerful assist in continuing my work as a Goodwill Ambassador for the National MS Society. I cherish the opportunities I have had to travel across the country bringing comfort to the many who are much less fortunate than myself and especially to have the opportunity to reach out to the 40 percent of MS patients not on therapy—who, due to fear or misconceptions, are not seeking drug treatment. I consider bringing attention to the latter group of utmost importance in my long-term objectives as a Goodwill Ambassador because MS continues its destruction on the

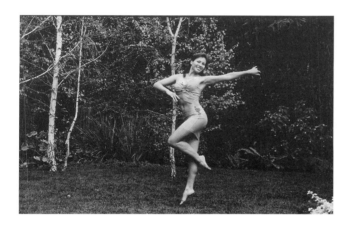

central nervous system even when you don't feel sick. New medications help to slow and reduce the damage, and may even help to repair it.

So, despite the trials I trust I am right where I belong, doing exactly what I am meant to be doing. I have learned that success is not simply a positive outcome; it is what you do with what is thrown your way in life, and I am living life to the fullest and passionately pursuing my dreams. I haven't had to and certainly don't intend on giving up on those dreams. I will be singing and dancing when I am ninety-five! For now, I know I am making a difference, eliciting smiles and sitting on top of the world.

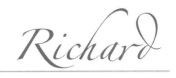

SIXTY-THREE

Editor's Note: Richard's wife Jennifer has taken the opportunity to write on Mr. Pryor's behalf.

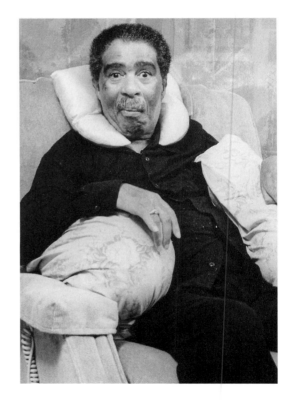

WHEN, AFTER A SEPARATION, Richard asked me, in 1994, to come back to Los Angeles and into his life again (which I never completely left), I had to think long and hard! Not only because of our tempestuous history but because the task he put before me was Herculean! Richard had been diagnosed with multiple sclerosis in 1986 and, since it is secondary progressive MS, he was deteriorating. As if that weren't enough, his personal life and business affairs were in need of immediate attention and rehabilitation as well. I would definitely have my work cut out for me! I was aware of the challenge and decided I might be able to help turn lemons into lemonade. And after all these years, Richard felt like family.

It is now nine years later and what a journey it has been! My life has been altered (not by Richard this time) and I have become well versed in the affairs of family court and other litigations. I have had a crash-course in business affairs, and have generally become a skilled administrator and CEO of a cottage industry! I have learned much about the medical field, more specifically MS, and the difficulties that accompany caregiving. But most of all, I view this time with Richard as a gift. MS is a cruel and determined disease but Richard fights everyday and still maintains a good quality of life, despite the harsh realities of a body under constant attack. We have left the past behind us and reclaimed the good and the love and the best of what we originally offered one another, before bad choices and cocaine intruded. We have even remarried. We laugh and

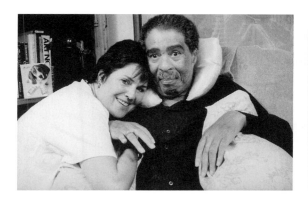 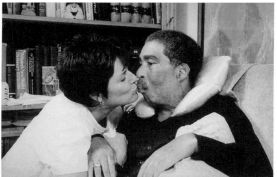

sometimes we cry. MS has in a strange way been a blessing. Perhaps it has even kept Richard alive. It has certainly made us grateful for the life we have now and has taught us to appreciate everyday that Richard is here. We both are amazed that he has survived and that we have been delivered to this time and place, together!

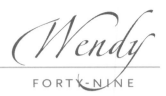
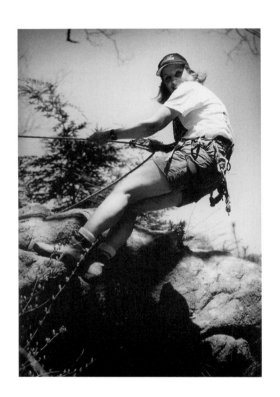

I WAS DIAGNOSED with remitting/relapsing multiple sclerosis in June of 1998. I was always a casual runner, running for exercise, mental therapy, and to be able to eat a lot and collect t-shirts. It was when returning from one of those runs that I noticed my left leg was numb. I ignored it for several months, figuring it was just another running injury that would eventually go away. A fall from a display window at work finally prompted me to seek medical help, which ultimately led to the diagnosis. It was running which not only led to the diagnosis, but became for me an outlet to overcome and cope with my MS. Despite the continued numbness and tingling, which I still have, I decided to see just how far and how hard I could push back at my MS. Without telling too many people, I decided to train for the Boston Marathon in the winter of 1999. My intention was to enter as an unofficial runner and see if I would be capable of running the 26.2 miles. About six weeks prior to the marathon, in February 2000, I changed my attitude and decided if that I was going to run, I wanted it to be official! I called the Multiple Sclerosis Society of Central New England to inquire if they had a number available.

I had no idea numbers were so coveted and hard to secure. In April 2000, I became #18,694! Life has never been the same since.

While beginning to train for my second marathon, in the fall of 2000, I heard about a man from Colorado who was talking about putting together a team of climbers with MS to climb Mt. McKinley. At first I didn't pay too much attention as I had never climbed before and knew that

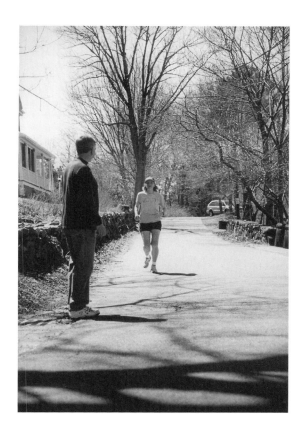

McKinley was a no-nonsense mountain for experienced mountaineers. But just like Boston 2000, I had to find out more. I eventually became the sole woman member on the seven man unguided team: Climb For The Cause, MS on Denali 2002.

A decision to climb a mountain such as McKinley when you are a forty-something wife and mother isn't yours alone to make. Following my husband's advice, I made a list of pros and cons. As the con list grew the pro list remained at three. It was due to those three very important reasons, however, that I accepted the challenge. The first and foremost was the mission of the climb, to show what people with MS are capable of and that a diagnosis of MS doesn't mean you have to give up your dreams. Second, we all wanted to encourage those newly diagnosed with MS to get on one of the available therapies as soon as possible, and third, I had my own personal reason. Never again in my life would I be offered such a challenge. The entire family was involved in the decision since they too would be greatly impacted by it. My husband, mother, and three boys all contributed to the success I had reaching the mountain. For the better part of a year I was away learning to climb on both the east and west coast. When I landed on that glacier, I was ready.

So many things come to mind when I think of the weeks spent on the mountain. The environ-

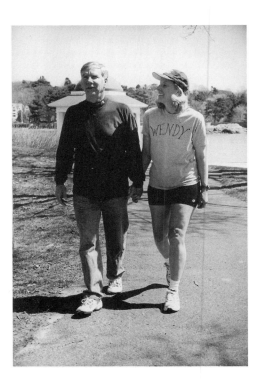

ment is harsh but very beautiful and always changing. One of the aspects that you can't train for or even know what to expect is life at altitude. Everything is harder because of the lack of oxygen in the air. The longer you are at altitude the more difficult life becomes—motivation, energy, clear thinking, and even eating and drinking can all be compromised. I often felt I would never be able to climb up or down again. Once you actually do start to move you regain most of your energy and motivation but the breathing is always difficult.

Still, despite everything, when I would stop and look around, I was always in awe as to where I was and how I came to get there. I still find it hard to believe that I was on the highest point in North America.

We climbed as high as the mountain would allow. It was very difficult to make the decision to turn back, which took us many days and attempts to make. Mountaineering is not defined by a summit, but more by gutting it out and staying with it as long as personal safety and conditions allow. We were successful on all counts but we were most successful because we fulfilled our mission, to show what people living with MS are capable of. We had the added challenge of climbing with a chronic disease and the added weight of carrying our daily injections. We were proud of our personal accomplishment on Denali but prouder still of why we did it in the first place and what it meant to us with MS and those newly diagnosed. Anytime I questioned my capabilities while climbing I would remind myself of the reason I wanted to climb Denali in the first place. My commitment to our mission and its message carried me along many times.

I can sum up my personal experiences in one word—gratitude. Gratitude that I was physically able to train for and climb Denali. Gratitude that I was afforded the opportunity to see something very few people ever see and experience. Gratitude that I was climbing for a cause so important and personally compelling to me. I hope that our climb and it's message will be an inspiration to someone newly diagnosed with MS and that they won't let that news discourage them from taking on a new challenge or giving up on something they enjoy.

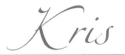

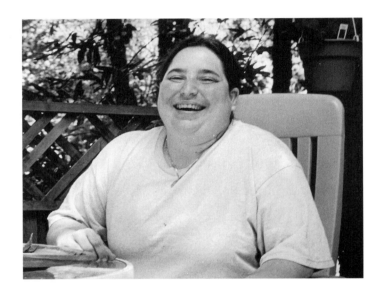

THIRTY-NINE

IT WAS THE WEEK of my twenty-eighth birthday when I was diagnosed with MS. I had a promising career in business management—very physical and very long hours. I loved it. A lot has changed since then.

I am now thirty-seven. To say that I have "settled in" with this disease would be a lie. The falling, dropping, confusion and problems with speech can be overwhelming at times. Especially all the "gee…you look fine!" comments, but life is good. Sometimes you have to make an effort to make it good, but life is still good.

For frustration I use a punching bag, which believe it or not helps a lot. Depression caused by this illness can pull you in if you let it.

Someday they will find a cure. Until then I will keep on smiling and looking forward to tomorrow. Get out and about, walk past your chair when you can. God bless, stay tough and don't *ever* give up.

Laurel

Kris is the love of my life. Kris and I had been together for two years when she was diagnosed with MS, it is now ten years later.

Communication is our best tool to use. Ups and downs are what I look to her for and she looks to me for, as a team we can't be beat.

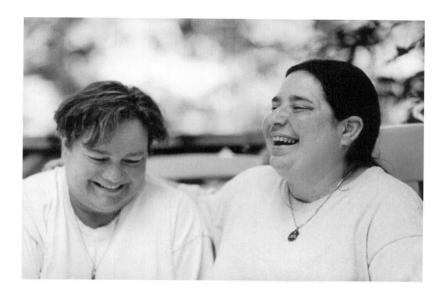

I lost both of my parents to cancer but MS is no better as a disease. With MS people look at you and think, "what's wrong with you?" It is hard to get any doctors to understand how one is feeling with MS. Kris and I have learned not to settle for less, and continue to search for that right doctor. It helps with your self-confidence.

There are times Kris and I need to push one another to get over the next molehill on the roller coaster ride of MS. We will continue to push each other, until the devastating statistics of MS fall.

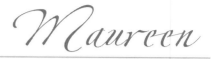
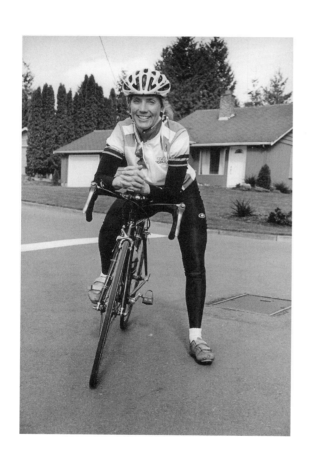

THIRTY-EIGHT

MULTIPLE SCLEROSIS came into my life when I was a member of the US Cycling Team in 1991. Through a lot of determination and hard work I was at the top of the sport. I had competed in World Championships, won National Championships, set a National Record, and earned many other honors. Then it all came crashing down. When racing in the Women's Tour de France my vision blurred so severely that I rode my bicycle off the road. What I didn't know then that I know now, is that I had ridden my bicycle off one road to begin a journey on another.

My world, as I knew it, had shattered. Everything I held to be meaningful *seemed* to be stripped away. With MS, I wondered how I could ever experience the joy, freedom, self-expression, drive and self-discovery that I so loved as a world-class cyclist. Meeting challenges was something I loved to do; it came naturally to me. This new challenge differed, however, in that it certainly was not one of my choosing. I came to real-

84

ize I might not have control over whether I cared to experience this challenge, but I did have control over my relationship to it and how I chose to grow through it.

With time, acceptance, education and exploration, I began to understand living an empowered life had less to do with what I could achieve, and more to do with who I am and how I choose to live my life. I came to know that I am constantly creating my life with my thoughts, ideas, expectations and actions. By continually working to align these things with the deepest part of who I am, I discovered that the qualities I so appreciated in myself as a world-class athlete had never been taken away. These are an expression of my spirit, which is boundless and can be express in so many ways.

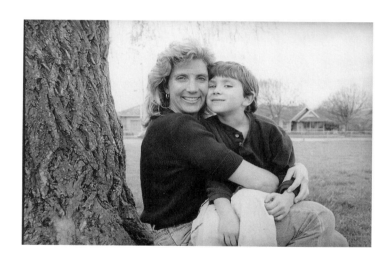

There's an old Buddhist saying, "fall down seven times, get up eight." When I first heard this, I thought, "Yes, that's it!" I've cried buckets of tears over this thing and shook my fists at the heavens more than once. By accessing whatever means necessary, I have managed to pick myself up, dust myself off, and get back to listening to my heart and following its guidance.

My pursuits within the past few years have included getting a Master's Degree in Integrated

Wellness, and establishing my own business as a motivational speaker, life coach and group facilitator. After losing my cycling career twelve years ago, I am back competing in a variety of cycling and athletic events. These are a few ways that I have been able to express, live and breathe what is meaningful to me.

Balancing being a single mother with self-care, work and recreation has been an adventure filled with triumphs and tribulations. My incredible love for my son and my intention to model for him what I feel is important in living a rich, full and empowered life is what guides me. He continually reminds me of what is the most important and real love.

I believe starting a course of treatment for MS six years ago, staying physically active, surrounding myself with a team of people who support and believe in me, practicing a variety of complementary medicines, and continuing to nurture and explore my connection with God and this great mystery called life, have all played an integral role in pulling me forward.

A year and a half after the diagnosis of MS I couldn't walk unaided. My vision at best had blurred so severely I couldn't function as a sighted person. I've experienced many challenges that have pushed me to the depth of my being. I've also experienced the wonders, magic and possibilities that life holds by continuing to explore, discover, embrace and embody the essence of what it means to be whole.

Jennifer

I remember first meeting Maureen about ten years ago in a Science of Mind class. I recall seeing different facets of her personality emerge as the weeks of the class progressed. These included a broad range of self- expression, from a raw power of belief in herself to shadowing doubts in her faith, expressions of vulnerability associated with health challenges and the tenacity of a champion where "failure is not an option," and an attitude that included a well educated respect for grounded scientific fact as well as a belief in the esoteric possibilities of metaphysics and magical dreams with fairytale endings. I knew I'd found a kindred spirit and the resonant connection between us grew from there.

She always sparks the courage and power within me by who she is being through all that she goes through. As our dear friend Doreen Palermo says, "Mo thrives in the impossible!" She thinks so big that it can humble the boldest of us. What I love is that she is the embodiment of a champion, without ever having to know the details of her background. It was much later that I learned of all she had accomplished as a professional athlete, and I was not surprised. She doesn't focus on the past, however; she uses the present moment to express her spirit.

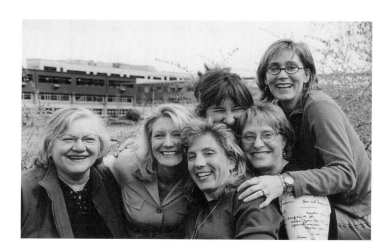

I admire how she gathers her resources, surrounds herself with loving friends, and never hesitates to ask for help when in need. She passionately shows up in full, whether on a high or a low. I've watched her grow through faith, and her acknowledgment that God shows up in all the faces around her. She is always in motion, whether in body or spirit, powering ahead like an eagle in purposeful flight, leaving a feather floating behind to remind us of the infinite possibilities available.

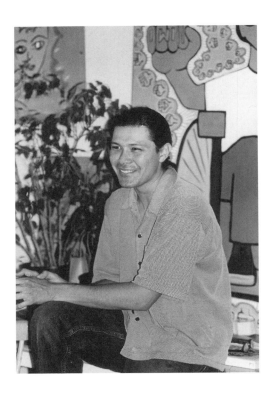

MULTIPLE SCLEROSIS is sobering challenge and a gift from above all wrapped up in one degenerative disease of the brain and nerves. It is certainly not much fun but, where there is pain and uncertainty, I am sure there is a message to be learned.

MS, in a way, is the only adult life I have known. I was fresh out of college and ready to take on the world when MS was presented to me as a way of life. The neurologist told me to hold off indefinitely on shopping for a wheelchair because MS can leave many folks able-bodied and only a small percent of patients get it severely.

For the most part the neurologist was correct. I have been diagnosed for eight years and I still can talk and smile as well as I always could. I do, however, need a cane most of the time to aid me in my walking and standing. My short-term memory has also been affected as remembering dates, schedules and names is an immediate impossibility.

For the most part, I can deal pretty well with the physical and cognitive symptoms but I do worry about how this disease will affect my family. I know that my family loves and supports me

88

but still I feel that this disease is something they really should not have to deal with. I would love to be able to handle all of this myself and know for sure that my family, especially my daughter, will not have to take too much responsibility for my current situation. With the last attack, I have learned that I cannot take on the entire burden alone and am grateful for my family to take the weight I am not able to hold. This disease has indeed brought a lesson of humbleness to me.

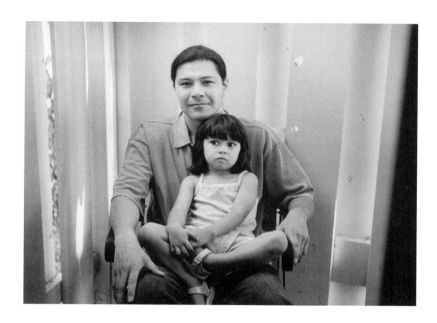

Even with all this change and uncertainty, I do feel that MS can be seen as a gift. I have always believed that people must make the best of what comes their way in life. With the diagnosis of MS, I was given at an early age the opportunity to test my belief. Now, I live that test on a day-to-day basis. That test constantly brings to mind the question of how I can keep my spirit intact even if a force greater than my choice can take my body and mind away.

The way I have dealt with the disease is through my ability and love for art. Recently, with the onset of new symptoms, I have compiled a large visual diary of what fears and questions came to mind during an attack of MS. I am now transferring these drawings to canvas so I can exhibit around the world what living through an attack of MS is like. MS has given me a subject that is personal, painful and world engaging. My art, painting and spiritual belief has given me the capability to channel pain and terrible uncertainty for a healing purpose and create at the same time a visual record of what it is to live with a diagnosis of MS.

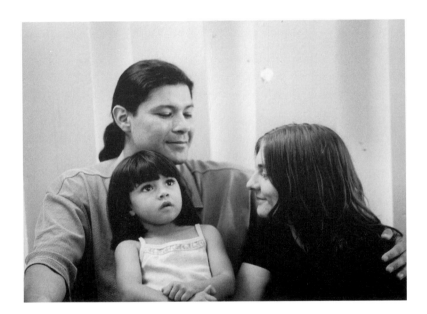

HEATHER

We all struggle with something. It's simple, right? At least, that is what I told myself the first six years of my relationship with Luis. Even after the disease revealed a glimpse of its gruesome potential, I failed to truly acknowledge it on a conscious level. I had been serving myself a potent cocktail of denial and detachment. I learned to cope, to stay focused and productive, to keep the ship afloat all the while—a drunkard behind the wheel.

I recall distinctly the moment a turbulent reality surged to the surface, breaking through my superficial calmness. Since life insists on maintaining balance, my calm naturally yielded to panic and I am still struggling to find a middle ground.

My experience with chronic illness as a wife and caregiver is both a loving burden and labored blessing. Someone told me that, "If you seek to learn patience, God will give you long lines to practice in." I sometimes think (mostly out of self-pity; so hard to admit) that I must have chosen the really hard lessons. But, I am blessed and humbled on my journey to find personal balance, to flow with the changing current, to love and live at this very moment, and breathe the spirit that is life. These are the treasures of the soul. It is so easy to fall back into "survival mode," thus neglecting our spirit. For the sake of those who are afflicted with acute or chronic illness—we, who love and care for those afflicted, must remember to add a little extra time in our day to seek our treasures.

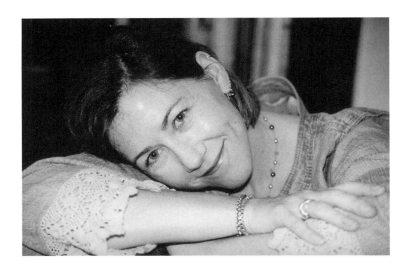

I REMEMBER SITTING on a cold, hard, wooden bench in my grammar school auditorium surrounded by uniformed class-mates, as well as all the other uniformed girls in the school. An announcement was made that there were forms available for anyone who wanted to partici-pate in a read-a-thon for multi-ple sclerosis. I picked a form up and noticed an illustration of a hound holding a magnifying glass in his paw, outlined in red. Next to the red hound were big, bold letters which stated: FIGHT MS. Not knowing what MS was, I took a form. I went around my neighborhood gathering signatures with promised pledges based on how many books I had read. Little did I know back then that one day, I too would be one of those people the red hound with the magnifying glass raised money for.

MS came knocking at my door just two months before my thirtieth birthday and just two months before my mother's death. What bad timing, although I don't think there ever is a good time to find out you have this disease.

MS has certainly changed my life forever. It will always be with me wherever I go and may affect me more severely. I think the hardest thing for me to face about having MS is the uncertainty of the future. The not knowing when or how it will next appear.

But, that same uncertainty has made me take a look at life. It has made me slow down and appreciate each day rather than trying to predict the future. I have had to learn to ask for help when I am unable to help myself, and have learned to accept help when it is given. I have had to learn to accept my life and to learn from it. Each day is a new day and every new person I meet has something to teach me.

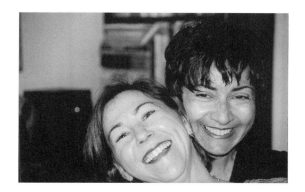 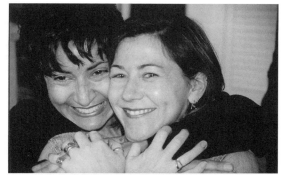

Embrace life; look at life straight on. Don't ever run from it because you never know whom you might meet or what lessons you might learn.

BONITA

It was not an easy decision to live with MS. I say this only because while I do have a choice in this matter, my partner does not.

I did not even think about "choice" at first. I did not think about MS or its effects on me because I was very, very busy taking care of Amelia and, at the same time, raising a teenager.

I had to withstand the pains. The pain of fear. The pain of disbelief. The pain of sorrow and the pain of loneliness.

And still get up in the morning to face the job that pays the bills.

It never gets easier, and it may never get better, but I will never regret my choice.

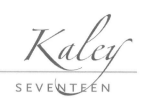
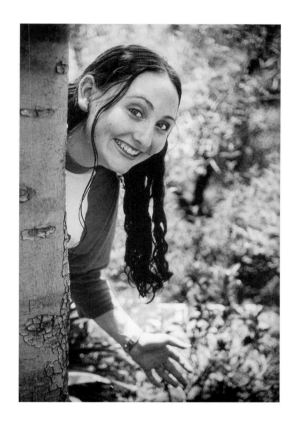

Tʜᴇʀᴇ ɪs ɴᴏ ʀᴀɪɴʙᴏᴡ without a storm. My storm hit when I was twelve years old and the diagnosis—multiple sclerosis. For three months I did not know what was wrong and doctors were reluctant to diagnose someone as young as myself with this disease. But finally it was definite and my life changed drastically—for the better. I changed everything about the way I lived my life and to this day, I do nothing the same way as I did it before. For me, being diagnosed was a wake up call. All of a sudden, I knew how lucky I was to be alive and to be able to walk, see and breathe each day. I learned that I could not take my health or my life for granted, especially the people in my life who have helped me every step of the way. My parents have always done everything in their power to take care of me and to make sure that I am taking care of myself. My brother Leor always keeps me laughing. When I was first diagnosed he kept my spirits up and he is always my sunshine in the rain.

It is probably because of him that I was able to stay so positive through the storm. I never asked, "why me" and was never angry at God. To this day I do not know how or why I was able to stay so optimistic and forge ahead with my life, but I am so thankful that I did. It did not take long for me to realize that my circumstances had altered my life and values, but that they had also affected the people around me. My friends began appreciating their lives and families more. They started enjoying life and living it to the fullest. I soon felt an instinct to share my story and tell the world

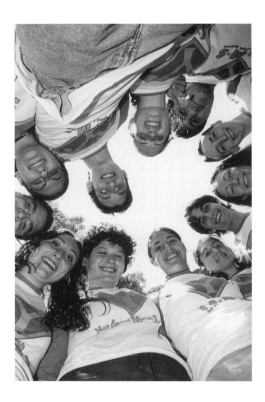

about my experiences so that others could learn from them. My friends and I agreed that not only did the general public not know enough about MS but that youth were especially uneducated about it. We all felt it was crucial that youth across the country know more about this disease.

And so my life purpose began. I started speaking to small groups of kids about my experiences and teaching about MS. I was soon speaking to groups of 800 teenagers at a time. We began raising money through the national MS Walk and today have raised over $100,000. In December of 2002 we founded our own nonprofit organization called YAMS, Inc—Youth Against Multiple Sclerosis. Our focus is twofold—to raise money for a cure and to spread awareness among youth. Today we have educated well over two thousand teens in greater Los Angeles as well as thousands

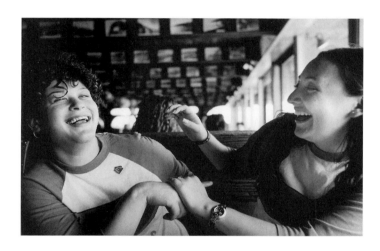

of teens all over the country. The greatest part is that YAMS is completely run by people under the age of eighteen.

I am now seventeen, and speaking to teenagers and sharing my story has been the most rewarding part of having MS. To be able to touch one person, to change one life is enough to get me out of bed each morning and to go to sleep each night satisfied that I have made a difference. The knowledge that a group of teenagers can change the world is truly unbelievable and empowering. What MS has taught me and the meaning it has filled my life with have been the rainbow throughout the storm. It has fulfilled my spirit and brought my life full circle. I know that there will always be sunshine through the rain. There are always showers here and there throughout the years and they always serve as a reminder to me of how fortunate I am and of why I am living today.

My friend Rona is also a reminder for me. She has been my best friend for eight years and has also grown with me through this MS experience. When I was diagnosed, I knew she could have seen having a friend with MS as a burden and walked away. Instead she was there for me more than ever before and has helped everyday since. When times get tough, she always reminds me of everything I have to be thankful for. She is always the level-headed one who helps make my goals concrete and my dreams come true. My vision to change the world and reach out to teenagers has become reality through my family, my friends, my community, God, and all that MS has taught me. MS has become a blessing rather than a curse and has truly shown me that there is no storm without a rainbow to follow.

Rona

Kaley and I are walking up the stairs at school. "I'm so proud of you! You doing okay?" I ask. "Hurts like hell, but I'll make it. This time," she says with a smile.

To many, it would seem unusual that a seventeen-year-old girl would be proud of her best friend for being able to walk up a flight of stairs. But this is what I have learned from having MS as a constant part of my life; unfortunately, this type of situation isn't unusual.

This was the first time in months that Kaley and I walked upstairs together in a place where elevators were available. Her current attack has been destroying her life, fiber by fiber, for the past year or so; her rights to control her legs, memory, attitude and other faculties were revoked by multiple sclerosis. Well, I once thought that health was a right. Once Kaley got MS, I realized that it is a privilege that many people don't have.

This was a hard lesson for the two of us to learn as little girls. Kaley was diagnosed with MS at the age of twelve, an experience that opened our eyes to the fact that weaknesses in health are real, even for a pre-teen girl. But we got over it, became stronger as friends and as people, and decided that we were going to do something about it. We understood that every aspect of life is precious, and were ready to take advantage of each opportunity in our lives to help others.

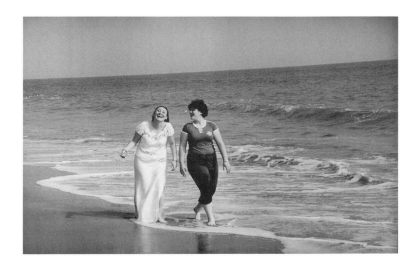

Wherever it came from, Kaley's strength was and is unwavering. Through the ups-and-downs of health and adolescent challenges, her powerful outlook on life is what keeps everyone fighting. It's amazing to see a teenager, who can't even stand up to make a speech at the kickoff event of our nonprofit organization, teach her audience about how much she still loves and appreciates life.

Her strength has been an inspiration to me. I have changed so much since Kaley got MS, and only for the better. I've learned from her that each person can make a big difference, and that anything you can imagine is possible. I've learned that life is really all about caring. Caring is the ultimate quick solution to living a good life. If you care about others, they'll care about you; if you care about the world, it will take care of you; if you care enough to learn how to fix the kitchen sink, you'll be able to repair it. I've learned that only by taking action may we reach our goals and show that we care. I've learned how to be a leader and take initiative, how to work with people, and how to give a little extra attention. I've gained something to fight for, something to be passionate about and spend my time working for. Learning how to prepare Kaley's daily injections even helped me in biology class! Dealing with MS, spreading awareness about it, and fundraising to find a cure are what really brought Kaley and me so close together, and continuously shape us into more sophisticated and grounded people.

I walked up those stairs again today at school, already almost winded from climbing the three previous flights. I thought to myself, "This is for Kaley," and I charged to the top of the steps. Today I climbed the stairs for her, but tomorrow she will be back again to climb them herself.

Jo

We have always believed that children are a blessing from God, Kaley is truly a blessing. She came to us bright-eyed and has led a life to be admired. Having MS has changed all our lives and has made us cherish her and each other every moment.

When she had her first symptoms, deep in my heart I truly did not think it was anything serious, it could not happen to us. Nothing serious could happen to my baby girl. My first fears arose as soon as we left the room after her MRI. I know that the technicians and nurses who worked there did not mean to let on, but they were just so kind, "you should take her for ice cream," one of them commented. I thought, "yeah, give her one more hour of blissful childhood before they tell us the bad news." She never did get that ice-cream or that last hour of blissful childhood before a neurologist that had observed her MRI soon insisted we come straight to his office. That's when things started to get scary for me.

I knew I had to be strong. As I thought it was nothing serious I had not even ask my husband to join us. The words, "there is some inflammation on her brain" will never leave me. Actually, I really wasn't too sure what he meant but it did sound serious. This was the beginning of my journey that I believe has brought out the best in each one of us.

From this experience I have seen so many loving qualities in my husband as a father. He developed this amazing relationship with Kaley; they could just spend hours together discussing life issues. He dealt with things in a very unique way, I saw through his quietness and realized that he had this strength that I did even know existed. He sought out the best doctors worldwide in order to find an accurate diagnosis. For Kaley this meant that her father would do anything in his power for her. They gained so much from each other. Through the way he dealt with this matter I learned that each one of us has our own approach to dealing with difficult circumstances.

Our other blessing, our son Leor, developed a very strong bond with Kaley, and their relationship has completely changed. Being able to laugh at some of the many difficult situations has helped all of us to cope better and he has especially helped Kaley. Instead of being a typical annoying little sibling, he has became a loving and caring brother to Kaley and a ray of sunshine for all of us. In a recent school essay, he wrote, "my sister has multiple sclerosis, she has taught me so many things about life. In my opinion, she was not born as a human, but as an angel of God to guide me through my life. My sister Kaley is my role model and though she has a chronic illness, she never ceases to amaze me." I found this amazing loving son through our experience with MS.

Like most mothers, I would trade places with Kaley and assume her disease in a heartbeat, but we all know that is not possible. My first call for help was to the National MS Society. This is where I learned that it would be possible to make it through this. I have learned just how precious life is and that we must cherish every moment we have together. I found in myself the strength that I did not know I had. I learned that we must educate ourselves and never stop fighting for a cure and that we must constantly be researching and learning about this disease in order to make a better life for the present and to find the cure that we need so imminently. I learned through talking with anyone and everyone about MS to be strong for Kaley and for all of us. This is what helps me get through this and gives me strength. I enjoy her, my life and family each day. I found that we have become closer as a family since we have needed each other so much; we have had to rely on each other, we did it, and continue to fight the fight every day. I found that you can turn the most painful experience in your life into something beautiful.

I know her friends, her teachers and who is important to her; if they are important to her then they are important to me. If I have a message to contribute to the world it would be to inspire other parents to stay positive, make a difference, appreciate your children, encourage them, listen to them, find their best qualities and the goodness in each of them, support them, and be with them. Learn to understand what they are all about as they are your blessings. Don't wait until you have time, make the time now. Appreciate every moment as we never know what tomorrow may bring.

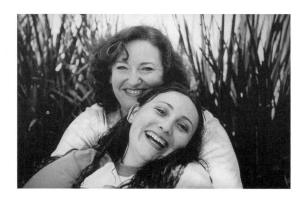
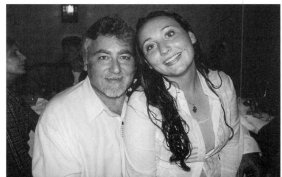

Dave

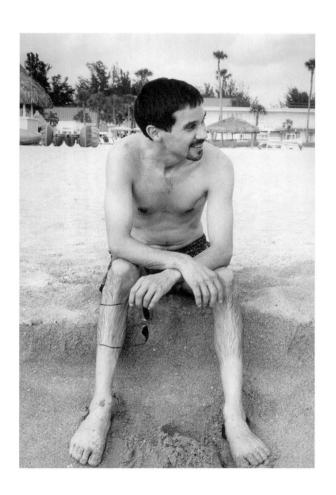

BEING DIAGNOSED with relapsing/remitting multiple sclerosis at the age of twenty-two was just the beginning. Being discharged from the Navy, near death from this disease, a divorce, and raising three children on my own were the icing on the cake.

It seems my life has been a series of transitions. During the first year of my MS I was very sick and in need of total care. I was in a wheelchair and totally paralyzed. After my MS went into remission two years later I was able to walk again with a cane—a situation that has remained stable to the present; however, I also faced the new heartbreak of a divorce and the responsibilities of assuming complete custody of three very young children. My kids have always been what has kept me going no matter what.

103

As they got older my role in their lives has changed. Not being needed as much, I had to look to projects outside the home to keep me busy. I started volunteering at the Greater Illinois Chapter of the National MS Society as an Information and Referral Specialist. It's very rewarding to talk to someone who is newly diagnosed and scared of what his or her future may bring. Knowing what it feels like when told, "You have MS," I can relate and give information on drug therapies available, local support groups to visit, and other valuable information.

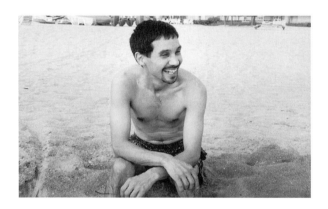

I've recently begun chairing a unique fundraiser, "Skydiving for MS." This began two years ago when I met a skydiver with MS at an MS related dinner who told me about the event, which had been loosely organized as a small, local fundraiser for the past three years. The challenge of assuming responsibility for this event piqued my interest and I've been hooked ever since. Within the past year our group has raised over $10,000 for the greater Illinois chapter of the National MS Society. Our organization has grown to include over two hundred members, thirty of which are people like myself who have MS and are skydiving. I know my limits physically and will accept when and if I get to the point I can no longer do this. Until then…

I often hear people say that MS has made them a better person. Personally, I feel MS has made me more aware of the wonderful people around me and I am very grateful for that.

Aㅤ FEW HOURS AGO, I was sitting on a hillside in West Virginia much too far away from the comfort of my boyfriend and my dogs back in Utah, and I was fighting back tears of frustration. After three grueling hours of riding, running and pushing my bike through thick mud and

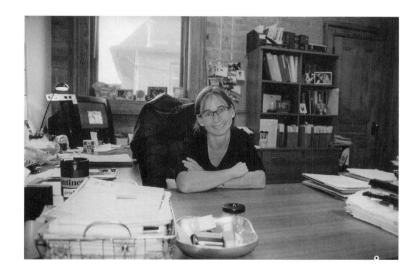

standing water, rocks, roots and trees, and getting well bruised and bloody in the process, I was tormented by self-doubt. I felt I had fallen well short of the lofty personal standards I had set for myself and was not fast enough, tough enough, good enough or deserving enough to compete as a mountain bike racer at the pro level. As I sat there fervently wishing for a hair shirt or some other

105

tool to punish myself for not having achieved a faster and better result, I ignored the reasons why I was there. Later, as I remembered those reasons, I regained some valuable perspective about why I push myself to such extremes, which are reflections I will take with me into the next challenge.

I was finally diagnosed with MS in the summer of 1996 after enduring six years of undefinable symptoms beginning in my first year of law school in Salt Lake City, Utah. I had always been involved in sports and since high school had coveted dreams of becoming an elite athlete. I had

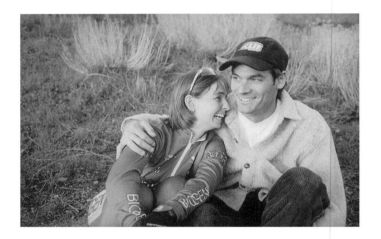

let those dreams fall by the wayside even before my diagnosis as I pursued my law career and adjusted to a new style of life in Utah. After my diagnosis and despite the set of hurdles my MS presented, including optic neuritis, seizures and partial paraplegia of my left side—my athletic aspirations came rushing back, and I began to pursue my cycling hobby in earnest. Given the unpredictability of MS, I did not want to look back and kick myself for not giving it all I had while I was still able. A year following my diagnosis, I was the very last person to qualify to compete in the 1997 Masters Worlds Championships in Switzerland—but qualify I did. Three years later, I turned pro. Since my diagnosis, I have opened up my own law practice specializing in employment discrimination, and I have had the opportunity to travel around North America to speak with groups of MS patients and healthcare providers about living and working with MS. However, it's likely I would neither have sought out nor had the courage to pursue those goals had I not become ill with MS. It is true that none of us would choose this illness. In reality, however, I consider my life the richer for it.

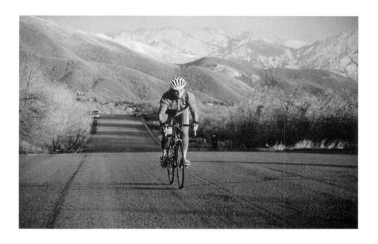

So, when I end up beating myself up for not being quite as fast, as strong or as deserving as I think I should be, I remind myself of my reasons for doing all of this. It is to show myself and others like me that indeed, we can rise to the challenge if we choose to do so—whatever that challenge may be. Much as this disease itself can fluctuate from day to day, so too may my own measure of success vary in meeting my goals. Some days success may mean winning the race. Yesterday, it just meant finishing it.

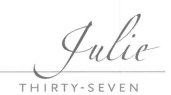

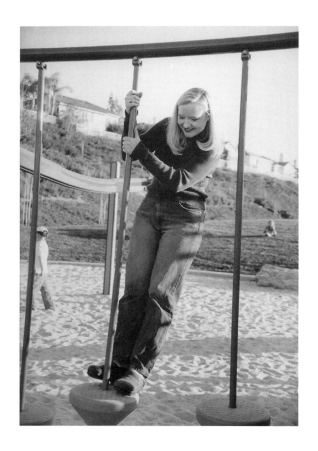

WHAT DOES HAVING MULTIPLE SCLE-ROSIS mean to me? Well, one of my favorite quotes is, "Survival means being born over and over." Each and every person is faced with some adversity in their life. How they choose to survive that adversity helps to define who they are. For me, challenges in my life have forced me to mature faster than I normally would have and given me a more meaningful, deeper life. In a strange way, I am grateful that MS gave me a wake-up call at a young age; it taught me to live my life to the fullest and to appreciate each day. Life is precious. Each day is a gift. Simplicity brings great happiness. How lucky I am that I didn't have to wait forty years to experience those epiphanies in old age.

Fourteen years ago, at twenty-three years of age, a diagnosis of relapsing-remitting MS was the beginning of a major transformation for me—physically, emotionally and spiritually. I spent the first part of my life as a "yes" person, a Type-A high achiever. The little things in life were less important than the drive to accomplish and more importantly, to please other people. With MS, I learned that taking care of myself had to come first. Honestly, I hated that! I will be the first to admit that it has been a hard adjustment, and I work at it each and every day. Fortunately, I have a remarkable husband who helps me to take life in stride and not sweat the small stuff.

Being diagnosed with a "disease" or having a disability is a strange thing. People begin to use that diagnosis or disability to define you and to make assumptions about your life. That can be frus-

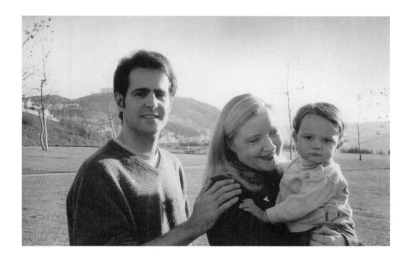

trating. A quote I love states, "We are all only temporarily able." A person may break their leg skiing, or fall off a curb and face injuries that completely change their lifestyle. My degree is in gerontology (the study of aging). I am frequently struck by the parallels older individuals often face that people with MS may face, including condescension and pity from others, identity transformation, stereotyping and prejudice, dependency, helplessness and frustration. But the parallels are not all negative. With aging and with MS, there can be enlightenment, reflection, appreciation for the simple things in life, pride, self-determination, spiritual growth, and an astonishing amount of love and support from others.

I am so fortunate to have many special friends and family members who have supported me on this journey with MS. However, my hero is my big brother, David. He has given his time, energy and money to fight MS for people everywhere. He is my biggest cheerleader in this journey; he gives me courage and hope, and is there to constantly remind me that although I may have MS, MS doesn't have me.

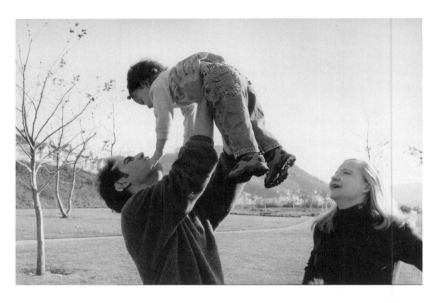

Margot
FORTY

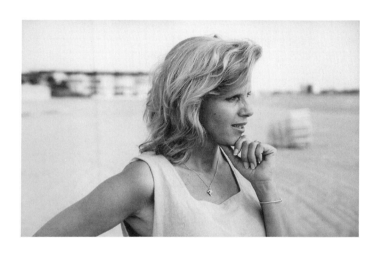

I'VE COME TO LOVE the study of footprints. I look to see where those who've gone before me have tread. When people are diagnosed with multiple sclerosis, where does the journey take them? I've climbed big hills and trudged through the woods for the answer. And this is what I've found: MS usually takes us to the fence that borders our own backyards. You can't go any further without knowing yourself.

Life is the journey, and MS is the train. It's not the view or my captain, but it takes me places, sometimes to the very core of my being. If I had taken the red train, I'd have seen different things. Life says, "This is the engine you'll be riding on," and off you go. Off you go on your own little journey, and you take yourself along the way. You take your fears, your dreams and struggles, pack them up and you go.

When I was diagnosed, I was due for an epiphany. I was standing at my backyard fence contemplating the leap. Where was my courage? I would find it some years later, delivered to my door by disease. And that's when I left my yard. Climbed right over the fence and found my way. MS gives ordinary people extraordinary strength.

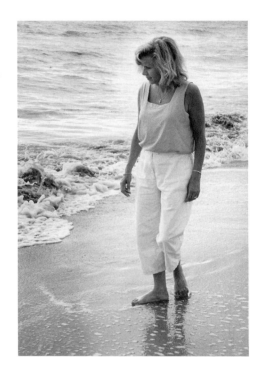 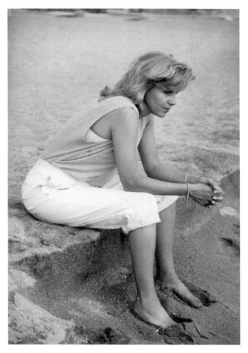

When I trace my own footsteps, I see where I've been. I remember the smile of a man in a wheelchair, the way he reached out and held my hand as I stood on able legs. I remember the love of a father, as he played football with his sons, not able to run anymore but able to love. And I think of the woman with MS who is holding her baby tonight, tempering her fears of the future and living for this moment alone. It's courage that I've witnessed and it's passion; passion to love and live no matter what, to make the best of what's been given and ride that invincible train. All the way to the end.

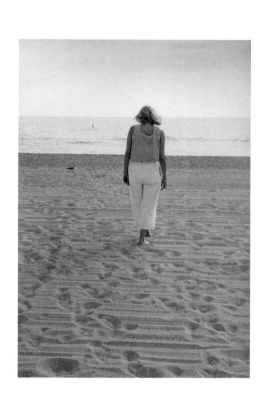